Contents

Acknowledgements

I would like to acknowledge and thank for the following people for their support in the writing of this book:

To my husband Mark for his considerable help and contributions, for his constant love and support and especially for inspiring and encouraging me to write this book; my parents Roy and Val for their positive encouragement and constant belief in my abilities; my dear friend Dee Chase for her valuable contributions and for her support and encouragement throughout the writing of this book; Dr Nathan Moss for his invaluable advice for Chapter 4 – Conditions of the Head, Neck and Shoulders; Carol Spencer and Sharon Holloway for kindly giving permission to publish their case studies, and finally to all the Indian Head Massage students at the Holistic Training Centre who have encouraged me to write this book. The publishers would like to thank Panos Pictures for permission to reproduce the photograph on page 2.

Preface

Originally developed as a family tradition in its native country of origin, Indian Head Massage has grown in popularity from being a technique which was mainly practised on the head by families in India, to become a comprehensive holistic therapy skill that addresses the widespread problems of stress in the western world. This book is designed for those undertaking a professional qualification in Indian Head Massage and addresses all the generic skills and knowledge required for commercial practice and competency in the workplace.

Indian Head Massage has grown in popularity in the late part of the 1990s to become an integral part of Holistic Therapy Course programmes in Further Education Colleges and Private Training Establishments. This book is presented in a workbook format in order to help students to generate sufficient evidence to reach a competent level for commercial practice. It is also formulated to assist tutors in their course design and delivery and in assessment of candidates' essential knowledge required for competency.

Helen McGuinness

Indian Head Massage:
Therapy Basics

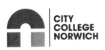

Orders: please contact Bookpoint Ltd, 130 Milton Park, Abingdon,
Oxon OX14 4SB. Telephone: (44) 01235 827720, Fax: (44) 01235 400454.
Lines are open from 9.00–6.00, Monday to Saturday, with a 24 hour message
answering service. You can also order from our website at www.hodderheadline.co.uk

British Library Cataloguing in Publication Data
A catalogue entry for this title is available from The British Library

ISBN 0 340 782 188

First published 2000
Impression number   14 13 12 11 10 9 8 7 6
Year   2004 2003

Typeset by Dorchester Typesetting Group Ltd.
Printed in Great Britain for Hodder & Stoughton Educational, a division of
Hodder Headline, 338 Euston Road, London NW1 3BH by
J. W. Arrowsmith Ltd, Bristol.

CHAPTER 1

Introduction to Indian Head Massage

Massage has always been an important feature of Indian family life. Indian Head Massage is a treatment that has evolved from traditional techniques that have been practised in India as part of a family ritual for over a thousand years.

Although the techniques are only applied to the upper part of the body (shoulders, upper arms, neck and head) collectively they represent a de-stressing programme for the whole body.

Traditional Indian Head Massage has many advantages in that it is
- non-invasive; the client remains fully clothed
- relatively quick to perform
- no special resources are needed
- special needs clients may receive treatment with the minimum fuss

By the end of this chapter you will be able to relate the following to your work as a holistic therapist:

> - The history and development of Indian Head Massage as a holistic therapy
> - The benefits and effects of Indian Head Massage

The history and development of Indian Head Massage

Ayurveda is recorded as the oldest Indian healing system. It is defined as the 'science of longevity' and is concerned with promoting positive health, beauty and long life. The early Ayurvedic texts date back nearly 4000 years and feature massage and the principles of holistic treatment, in that health results from harmony within one's self. The Ayurvedic view of health is in physical, emotional and spiritual well being and that health is maintained by the balance of three subtle life-giving forces or doshas:

- **VATA**: a comibination of Air and Ether. It is responsible for all movements of the mind, body and senses, and the process of elimination. The unique characteristic of Vata is dryness

- **PITTA:** is a combination of Fire and Water. It is responsible for heat, energy, metabolism and digestive functions of the body. The unique characteristic of Pitta is heat
- **KAPHA:** is a combination of Earth and Water. It is responsible for physical stability, proper body structure and fluid balance. The unique characteristic of Kapha is heaviness

The Hindus used techniques preserved in the Sanskrit texts 2,500 years ago, which detail the underlying principles of Ayurveda in maintaining balance in the body and a healthy balance of doshas.

Traditionally, massage has always been an important feature of family life across the generations. In India, it is customary for babies to be massaged every day from birth and to be massaged continually until they are 3 years old. From the age of 6 they are taught to show love and respect by sharing a massage with family members.

It is considered compulsory for a bride and groom to receive a massage with chemicals and oils before marriage. This ceremonial massage is considered to help relax the bride and groom, give them stamina and psychic strength, as well as promote health and fertility. In India, it is also tradition to massage expectant mothers to help them cope with the physical and emotional demands of labour; massage is applied daily for a minimum of 40 days after the birth. Weekly massage is a family event in India and for the majority continues throughout life to old age.

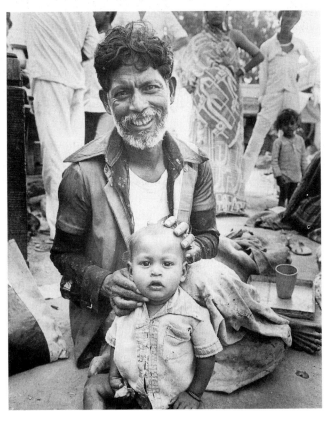

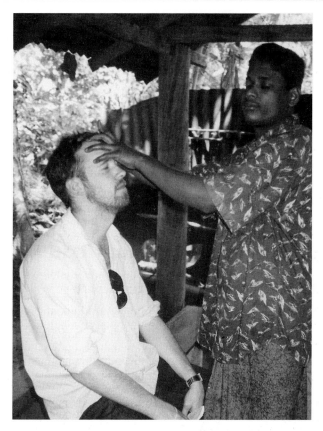

The Indian Head Massage techniques practised today have originally evolved from traditional rituals of Indian family grooming. Over generations, Indian women have been taught by their mothers to massage different oils such as coconut, sesame, olive, almond, herbal oils, buttermilk, mustard oil and henna into their scalp in order to maintain their hair in a beautiful condition.

In India barbers have developed a more stimulating and invigorating head massage to incorporate into their daily treatments and this has been passed down through the generations from barber father to barber son. The original tradition of Indian Head Massage has therefore been passed on through the family generations, as Indian women have been taught the tradition of hair massage and grooming from their mothers and barbers' sons have learnt techniques from their fathers.

In India, head massage forms an integral part of family life and is often a ritual that is performed not only at home within families but is commonly seen being performed on street corners, the beach and in barbers' shops. Although Indian Head Massage has been in existence in India for many years, it has only recently started to gain popularity in the West.

Today, Indian Head Massage is no longer confined only to the head area and has been westernised to include treating other parts of the body vulnerable to stress such as the neck, upper arms and shoulders. It is important to realise that there is an integral relationship between the head, neck, shoulders and upper arms, and by incorporating these parts the treatment becomes more of a stress management treatment, rather than a treatment just designed to stimulate the head and improve the hair growth and condition.

Indian Head Massage is today one of the fastest growing holistic therapies as it opens out a different market to holistic therapists.

Clients seeking relief from stress and tension are often embarrassed about removing their clothing or they have daily constraints in their life such as time. The strengths of Indian Head Massage lie in the fact that the client remain fully clothed, and that it can be performed anywhere. It is also quick to apply and extremely effective in term of results.

The Benefits and Effects of Indian Head Massage

Although the techniques involved in Indian Head Massage involve only the upper part of the body, the potential benefits are widespread. It can be said that Indian Head Massage is a truly holistic therapy in that it has many physiological and psychological benefits; many clients comment on the fact that they feel as if their whole body is balanced after the treatment.

EFFECTS	BENEFITS
Increase in blood flow to the head, neck and shoulders	■ Nourishes the tissues and encourages healing ■ Improves the circulation; the delivery of oxygen and nutrients is improved via the arterial circulation and the removal of wastes is hastened via the venous flow.
Increased lymphatic flow to the head, neck and shoulders	■ Aids the elimination of accumulated toxins and waste products ■ Reduces oedema ■ Stimulates immunity
Relaxes the muscle and nerve fibres of the head, neck and shoulders	■ Relieves muscular tension and fatigue ■ Increases flexibility ■ Improves posture ■ Can help to relieve tension headaches and aches and pains

EFFECTS	BENEFITS
Reduces spasms, restrictions and adhesions in the muscle fibres	■ Relieves pain and discomfort ■ Improves joint mobility
Decreases inflammation in the tissues	■ Pain relief ■ Reduces stress placed on bones and joints
Decreases stimulation of the sympathetic nervous system	■ Slows down and deepens breathing ■ Slows down the heart rate ■ Helps reduce blood pressure ■ Reduces stress and anxiety
Activates the parasympathetic nervous system	■ Encourages the body to rest and relax ■ Helps promote sleep
Improves circulation to the skin and the hair	■ Encourages cell regeneration
Increases circulation to the scalp	■ Promotes healthy hair growth ■ Helps improve the condition of the skin and hair
Relaxes and soothes tense eye muscles	■ Helps relieve tired eyes and eyestrain ■ Brightens the eyes
Increases the supply of oxygen to the brain	■ Helps relieve mental fatigue ■ Promotes clearer thinking ■ Improves concentration ■ Increases productivity
Stimulates the release of endorphins from the brain	■ Helps relieve pain ■ Helps relieve emotional stress and repressed feelings ■ Elevates the mood – can help anxiety and depression
Encourages the release of stagnant energy and restores the energy flow to the body	■ Creates a feeling of balance and calm

Self Assessment Questions

1) What is Indian Head Massage ?

2) Give a brief outline of how Indian Head Massage has evolved

3) List 5 physical benefits of Indian Head Massage

4) List 3 psychological benefits of Indian Head Massage

CHAPTER 2

Essential Anatomy & Physiology for Indian Head Massage

In order to understand the physiological effects of Indian Head Massage on the body, it is important for holistic therapists to have knowledge of essential anatomy and physiology in order to carry out treatments safely and effectively. This chapter is devoted to the anatomy and physiology relevant to Indian Head Massage in relation to the areas directly affected by the treatment.

By the end of this chapter you will be able to relate the following knowledge to your practice in Indian Head Massage:

- The structure and functions of the skin and hair
- The bones of the shoulder, neck, upper arm, skull and face
- The muscles in relation to the shoulders, neck, upper arms, scalp and face
- The blood flow to and from the head and neck
- The lymphatic drainage of the head and neck
- The nerve supply to the head and neck
- The mechanism of respiration

The Skin

The skin is the largest organ of the body and provides the therapeutic foundation for treatment.

- Each client's skin varies in its colour, texture and condition.
- A client's skin can reflect their physiological as well as psychological state and it is through touch that therapists can help to evaluate this information.

■ Physiological signs on the skin may be shown by the client's colour and circulation, whereas physiological status may be reflected by muscular tightness. How clients feel about themselves and about others is often reflected in the skin (clients who are anxious may be hot and sweaty) Therapists can gather this important information through therapeutic touch.

A thorough knowledge of the structure and functions of the skin will help the therapist to treat clients more effectively. There are two main layers of the skin:
■ The epidermis which is the outer thinner layer
■ The dermis which is the inner thicker layer

Below the dermis is the subcutaneous layer which attaches to organs and tissues.

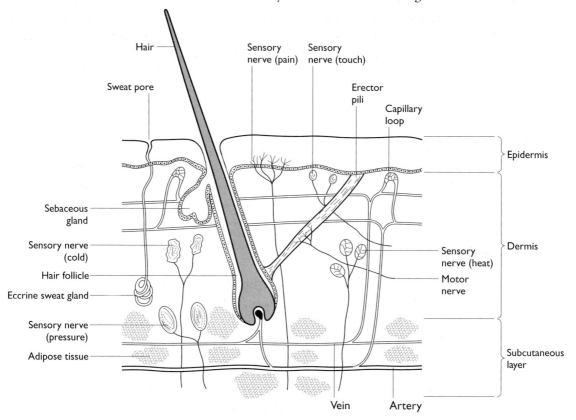

THE EPIDERMIS

The epidermis is the most superficial layer of the skin and consists of five layers of cells:
■ the horny layer – outermost layer
■ the clear layer
■ the granular layer
■ the prickle cell layer

- the basal cell layer – innermost layer
- The three outermost layers (horny, clear and granular) consist of dead cells as a result of the process of keratinisation. The cells in the very outermost layer are dead and scaly and are constantly being rubbed away by friction.
- The inner two layers are composed of living cells.
- The epidermis does not have a system of blood vessels, therefore all nutrients pass into the cells of the epidermis from blood vessels in the deeper dermis.

The Basal Cell Layer

This is the deepest of the five layers. It consists of a single layer of column cells on a basement membrane which separates the epidermis from the dermis. In this layer the new epidermal cells are constantly being reproduced. These cells last about six weeks from reproduction before being discarded into the horny layer. New cells are therefore formed by division, pushing adjacent cells towards the skin's surface. At intervals between the column cells which divide to reproduce, are the large star-shaped cells called melanocytes which form the pigment melanin, the skin's main colouring agent.

Prickle Cell Layer

This is known as the prickle cell layer because each of the rounded cells contained within it have short projections which make contact with the neighbouring cells and give them a prickly appearance. This living cells of this layer are capable of dividing by the process mitosis.

Granular Layer

This layer consists of distinctly shaped cells, containing a number of granules which are involved in the hardening of the cells by the process known as keratinisation. This layer links the living cells of the epidermis to the dead cells above.

Clear Layer

This layer consists of transparent cells which permit light to pass through. It consists of three or four rows of flat dead cells which are completely filled with keratin; they have no nuclei as the cells have undergone mitosis. The clear layer is very shallow in facial skin but thick on the soles of the feet and the palms of the hands and is generally absent in hairy skin.

Horny Layer

This is the most superficial outer layer, consisting of dead, flattened keratinised cells which have taken approximately a month to travel form the basal cell layer. This outer layer of dead cells is continually being shed, this process is known as desquamation.

Cell regeneration

Cell regeneration occurs in the epidermis by the process mitosis. It takes approximately a month for a new cell to complete its journey from the basal cell layer where it is reproduced to the granular layer where it becomes keratinised, to the horny layer where it is desquamated.

The Dermis

The dermis lies below the epidermis and is the deeper layer of the skin. Its key functions are to provide nourishment to the epidermis and to give a supporting framework to the tissues.

The dermis has two layers: a superficial papillary layer and a deeper reticular layer. The superficial papillary layer is made up of fatty connective tissue and is connected to the underside of the epidermis by cone-shaped projections called dermal papillae which contain nerve endings and a network of blood and lymphatic capillaries. The deeper reticular layer is formed of tough fibrous connective tissue which contains the following:

- collagen fibres which help to give the skin strength and resilience
- elastic fibres which help to give the skin elasticity
- reticular fibres which help to support and hold all structures in place

Cells present in the dermis include

- mast cells which secrete histamine (involved in allergies) causing dilation of blood vessels to bring blood to the area
- phagocytic cells, which are white blood cells that are able to travel around the dermis destroying foreign matter and bacteria
- fibroblasts, which are cells that help form new fibrous tissue

Blood Supply

Unlike the epidermis the dermis has an abundant supply of blood vessels which run through the dermis and the subcutaneous layer.

Arteries carry oxygenated blood to the skin via arterioles ands these enter the dermis from below and branch into a network of capillaries around active or growing structures. These capillary networks form in the dermal papillae to provide the basal cell layer of the epidermis with food and oxygen. They also surround the sweat glands and erector pili muscles, two appendages of the skin.

The capillary networks drain into venules, small veins which carry the deoxygenated blood away from the skin and remove waste products. The dermis is therefore well supplied with capillary blood vessels to bring nutrients and oxygen to the germinating cells in the basal cell layer of the epidermis and to remove waste products from them.

Lymph Vessels

There are numerous lymphatic vessels in the dermis. They form a network in the dermis facilitating the removal of waste form the skin's tissue. The lymphatic vessels in the skin generally follow the course of veins and are found around the dermal papillae, glands and hair follicles.

Nerves

There is a wide distribution of nerves throughout the dermis. Most nerves in the skin are sensory, which send signals to the brain and are sensitive to heat, cold, pain, pressure and touch. The dermis also has motor nerves which relay impulses to the brain and are responsible for the dilation and constriction of blood vessels, the secretion of perspiration from the sweat glands and the contraction of the erector pili muscles attached to hair follicles.

The Subcutaneous Layer

This is a thick layer of connective tissue found below the dermis. The type of tissue found in this layer (areolar and adipose) help support delicate structures such as blood vessels and nerve endings.

The subcutaneous layer contains the same collagen and elastin fibres as the dermis and contains the major arteries and veins which supply the skin and form a network throughout the dermis. The fat cells contained within this layer help to insulate the body by reducing heat loss. Below the subcutaneous layer lies the subdermal muscle layer.

FACTORS AFFECTING THE SKIN

DIET – a healthy body is needed for a healthy skin. The skin can be thought of as a barometer of the body's general health.

VITAMIN A: helps repair the body's tissues and helps prevent dryness and ageing

VITAMIN B: helps improve the circulation and the skin's colour, and is essential to cellular oxidation

VITAMIN C: is essential for healing and to maintain levels of collagen in the skin

WATER – drinking an adequate amount of water (approximately 6-8 glasses per day) aids the digestive system and helps to prevent a build up of toxicity in the tissues of the skin.

SLEEP – sleep is essential to physical and emotional well-being and is one of the most effective regenerators for the skin.

STRESS AND TENSION – when the body is subjected to regular stress and tension it can cause sensitivity and allergies in the skin as well as encourage the formation of lines around the eyes and the mouth.

EXERCISE – regular exercise promotes good circulation and increased oxygen intake and blood flow to the skin.

ALCOHOL – alcohol has a dehydrating effect on the skin and excess consumption causes the blood vessels in the skin to dilate.

SMOKING – smoking affects the skin's cells and destroys vitamins B and C which are important for a healthy skin. Smoking dulls the skin by polluting the pores and increases the formation of lines around the eyes and the mouth.

MEDICATION – medication can affect the skin by causing dehydration, or sensitivity and/or allergies.

HORMONES – the natural glandular changes of the body have an effect on the condition of the skin throughout life.

- During puberty, the sex hormones stimulate the sebaceous glands which may cause some imbalance in the skin.
- At the onset of menstruation the skin may erupt due to the adjustment of hormone levels at that time.
- During pregnancy, pigmentation changes may occur, but usually disappear at birth.
- During the menopause the activity of the sebaceous glands is reduced and the skin becomes drier.

AGE – the natural process of ageing naturally affects the skin. From the mid thirties the skin starts to lose its firmness and fine lines and wrinkles start to appear. In the forties and fifties lines and wrinkles will deepen and loss of muscle tone causes sagging of the skin on the cheeks and the neck. The connective tissue in the skin loses its elasticity and becomes less firm, and the skin becomes thinner and finer. As part of the ageing process the process of cell regeneration in the skin decreases and the skin appears dry and dull.

APPENDAGES OF THE SKIN

The appendages are accessory structures that lie in the dermis of the skin and project onto the surface through the epidermis. These include the hair, the erector pili muscle, sweat and sebaceous glands.

The Hair

Hair is an appendage of the skin which grows from a sac-like depression in the epidermis called a hair follicle. Hair grows all over the body, with the exception of the palms of the hands and the

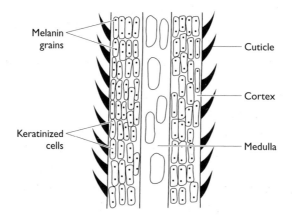

Melanin grains

Keratinized cells

Cuticle

Cortex

Medulla

soles of the feet. The primary function of a hair is physical protection. For example, the hair on the scalp provides partial shading from the suns rays, and the hairs in the nostrils, eyelashes and eyebrows provide protection from foreign particles.

The Structure of a Hair

The hair is composed mainly of the protein keratin and is therefore a dead structure. Longitudinally the hair is divided into three parts:

- **HAIR SHAFT** – the part of the hair that lies above the surface of the skin
- **HAIR ROOT** – the part of the hair which is found below the skin
- **HAIR BULB** – the enlarged part at the base of the hair root

Internally the hair has three layers which all develop from the matrix, which is the active growing part of the hair.

CUTICLE: this is the outer layer and is made up of transparent protective scales which overlap one another. The cuticle protects the cortex and gives the hair its elasticity.

CORTEX: this is the middle layer and is made up of tightly packed keratinised cells containing the pigment melanin, which gives the hair its colour. The cortex helps to give strength to the hair.

MEDULLA: this is the inner layer and is made up of loosely connected keratinised cells and tiny air spaces. The layer of the hair determines the sheen and colour of the hair due to the reflection of light through the air spaces.

Hair Growth

Hair growth originates from the central area of the hair bulb, the matrix, which is the active growing area where the hair cells divide and reproduce. The living cells produced in the matrix are then pushed upwards from their source of nutrition and are converted to keratin to produce a hair that eventually projects from the open end of the follicle.

The Growth Cycle of the Hair

Hair has a growth pattern which ranges from approximately four to five months for an eyelash hair to approximately four to seven years for a scalp hair.

At the end of each hair's life span, the root of the hair separates from its matrix and remains in the follicle until it falls out or is pulled out. The follicle then shrinks and enters a period of rest. Following its rest period, the follicle will either degenerate completely or enlarge to form a new hair bulb and produce another hair.

Factors Affecting Hair Growth

The way our hair looks has a great impact on the way we feel. Shiny lustrous hair is synonymous with good health and vitality. Factors such as diet, age and hormones directly determine its appearance.

DIET – health of the hair comes from within and therefore a poor diet can affect the condition of the hair. For healthy hair, it is important to have a diet rich in protein, essential fatty acids, vitamin B complex and C help provide nourishment for hair follicles.

- Minerals such as iron, sulphur and zinc can help the hair if the important mineral content of the hair is missing and the hair is dull in appearance.
- Vitamin B5 is important to help relieve stress in the hair and Vitamin A is useful for a dry and scaly scalp.

ILLNESS – prolonged illness and stress can cause both hair loss and greying, due to the fact that the body is starved of essential nutrients and cell metabolism is slowed down due to infection and /or disease.

HORMONAL INFLUENCES – the hair is often affected by hormonal changes occurring in the body such as puberty, pregnancy and the menopause. Hair can become more greasy during menstruation. It may become dry due to a thyroid problem or there may be a temporary hair loss during pregnancy (especially after delivery). A drop in oestrogen during the menopause can have a profound effect on the hair, causing it to become dry, coarse and brittle.

OVER PROCESSING – perming and dyeing the hair can alter the shaft of the hair often making it dry and brittle. Frequent use of shampoos full of detergents and chemicals can also dry out the scalp.

STRESS AND TENSION – tension in the scalp can reduce the circulation of oxygen and starve the hair root of nutrients needed for healthy growth.

SHOCK – shock has been known to cause the hair to fall out.

MEDICATION – medication can affect the hair by drying the skin which in turn blocks the follicles with dead keratinised cells which block the circulation to the scalp.

ALLERGIES – reaction to products used on the hair and scalp may cause sensitisation of the scalp and this affect the circulation of blood to the hair. Some clients may develop dandruff in response to sensitisation of hair products.

Hair Colour

Hair colour is due to the presence of melanin in the cortex and medulla of the hair shaft. In addition to the standard black colour, the melanocytes in the hair bulb produce two colour variations of melanin, brown and yellow. Blond, light coloured and red has a high proportion of the yellow variant. Brown and black hair possesses more of the brown and black melanin.

> **KEY NOTE** Hair turns grey when the melanocytes in the hair bulb stop producing melanin.

Erector Pili Muscle

This is a small smooth muscle which is attached at an angle to the base of a hair follicle, which serves to make the hair stand erect in response to cold.

Sweat glands

There are two types of sweat glands; the majority are called eccrine glands which are simple coiled tubular glands that open directly onto the surface of the skin. There are several million of them distributed over the surface of the skin but are most numerous in the palms of the hands and the soles of the feet.

Their function is to regulate body temperature and help eliminate waste products. Their active secretion sweat is under the control of the sympathetic nervous system.

The other type of sweat glands are called apocrine glands; these are connected with hair follicles and are only found in the genital and underarm regions. They produce a fatty secretion; breakdown of the secretion by bacteria leads to body odour.

Sebaceous Glands

These glands are found all over the body, except for the soles of the feet and the palms of the hands. They are more numerous on the scalp, face, chest and back.

Sebaceous glands commonly open into a hair follicle but some open onto the skin surface. They produce an oily substance called sebum which contains fats, cholesterol and cellular debris.

Sebum coats the surface of the skin and the hair shafts where it prevents excess water loss, lubricates and softens the horny layer of the epidermis and softens the hair.

FUNCTIONS OF THE SKIN

Protection

The skin acts like a physical barrier protecting the underlying tissues from abrasion. Keratin, a protein found in the skin provides protection by waterproofing the skin's surface, helping to keep water in and out. The skin also provides limited protection from ultra violet radiation through specialised cells called melanocytes found in the basal cell layer of the epidermis. The skin's acidic secretions (sweat and sebum), known as the acid mantle act as an barrier against foreign agents such as bacteria and viruses.

Sensation

The skin is like an extension of the nervous system in that it receives stimuli such as pressure, pain and temperature from the external environment and brings this information to the central nervous system.

Heat Regulation

The skin helps to regulate the body temperature's at a temperature of 37°C. When the body is losing too much heat, the blood capillaries near the skins surface constrict to keep warmth in and closer to major organs.

When the body is too warm, the blood capillaries dilate to allow more blood to flow near the surface in order to cool the body; the sweat glands also help to cool the body down through the production of sweat.

Excretion

The skin functions as a minor excretory system, eliminating waste through perspiration.

Secretion

The specialised glands in the skin called the sebaceous glands secrete the oily substance sebum which flows onto the skins surface, lubricating it and keeping it soft and pliable.

Absorption

The skin has limited absorption properties. Substances that can be absorbed by the epidermis are fat-soluble substances such as oxygen, carbon dioxide, fat-soluble vitamins, steroids and essential oils.

Vitamin D production

Located in the skin are molecules that are converted by the ultra violet rays in sunlight to vitamin D. The vitamin D produced is then absorbed into the blood vessels and used by the body for the maintenance of bones and the absorption of calcium and phosphorus in the diet.

> **KEY NOTE** Indian Head Massage can help to bring about an improvement in a client's skin and hair condition over a period of time. The increased circulation to the skin can increase cell nutrition and regeneration, as well as increase elimination of waste from the skin's tissues. Dead keratinised cells which are blocking the pores of the skin can be loosened by massage and the blood supply can flow more freely to feed the skin and hair with nutrients. Indian Head Massage can also help to increase the production of sebum from the sebaceous glands, helping to lubricate the skin and hair and improve its condition.

The Skeleton

The skeleton is the structure and framework on which other body systems depend for support and protection. It is therefore the physical foundation of the body. The main functions of the skeleton are to provide a means of protection, support and attachment for muscles. The skeleton is very important to a therapist as it provides landmarks for locating muscles.

The areas treated with Indian Head Massage include the shoulders, neck, upper arms and head which all have an integral relationship, and these are discussed in order for a therapist to have a knowledge of the regional anatomy they are working on.

THE BONES OF THE SHOULDERS

The shoulder girdle connects the upper limbs with the thorax and consist of 4 bones:

- Two clavicles
- Two scapulae

The **CLAVICLE** forms the anterior part of the shoulder girdle. It is a long slender bone with a double curve which is located at the base of the neck and runs horizontally between the sternum and the shoulders.

It articulates with the sternum at its medial end and the scapula at its lateral end.

The clavicle acts as a brace for the scapula, helping to hold the shoulders in place.

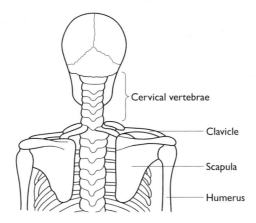

Cervical vertebrae

Clavicle

Scapula

Humerus

The **SCAPULAE** form the posterior part of the shoulder girdle and are located on either side of the upper back. The scapula is a large flat bone triangular in outline, which articulates with the clavicle and the humerus. The scapula has several prominent processes that serve as attachments for muscles and ligaments. The combined action of scapula, clavicle, humerus and associated muscles allows for a considerable amount of movement of the shoulder and upper limbs.

THE BONES OF THE NECK

The neck comprises of seven bones known as the cervical vertebrae. Although they are the smallest vertebrae in the spine their bone tissue is denser than those in any other region of the vertebral column.

The top two cervical vertebrae are named:

C1 is called the **ATLAS** and is the bone that sits at the top of the vertebral column embedded in the base of the skull. The atlas supports and balances the head. Sliding joints on either side of the atlas allow the head to move up and down.

C2 is called the **AXIS** which has a peg-like hook that fits into a notch in the atlas. The ring and peg structure of the atlas and axis allows for movement of the head from side to side.

- The transverse processes of the cervical vertebrae are distinctive in that they have transverse foramina (or holes) which serve as passageways for arteries leading to the brain.
- The spinous processes of the second through to the fifth cervical vertebrae are uniquely forked to provide attachment for the elaborate lattice of muscles of the neck.
- The spinous process of the seventh cervical vertebrae is longer and can be felt through the skin as it protrudes beyond the other cervical spines.

THE BONES OF THE UPPER ARM

The humerus is the long bone of the upper arm and is the largest bone of the upper extremity. The head of the humerus bone articulates with the scapula to form the shoulder joint and the distal end of the bone joints with the radius and ulna (bones of the forearm) to form the elbow joint.

THE SKULL

The skull rests upon the upper end of the vertebral column and weighs around eleven pounds! It consists of 22 bones; eight bones that make up the cranium and thirteen forming the facial skeleton.

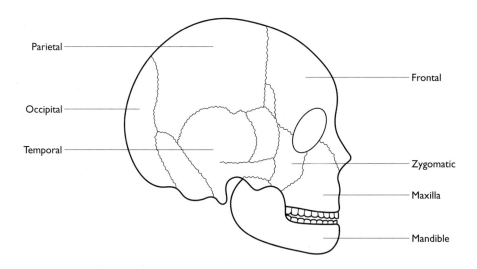

The Cranium encloses and protects the brain and provides a surface attachment for various muscles of the skull. The eight bones of the cranium are as follows:

- One **FRONTAL** bone forms the anterior part of the roof of the skull, the forehead and the upper part of the orbits or eye sockets. Within the frontal bones are the two frontal sinuses one above each eye near the midline

- Two **PARIETAL** bones form the upper sides of the skull and the back of the roof of the skull
- Two **TEMPORAL** bones form the sides of the skull below the parietal and above and around the ears. The temporal bone contributes to part of the cheekbone via the zygomatic arch (formed by the zygomatic and temporal bones)
- Located behind the ear and below the line of the temporal bones are the mastoid processes to which the stermomastoid muscles of the neck are attached
- One **SPHENOID** bone which is located in front of the temporal bone and serves as a bridge between the cranium and the facial bones. It articulates with the frontal, temporal, occipital and ethmoid bones.
- One **ETHMOID** bone which forms part of the wall of the orbit, the roof of the nasal cavity and part of the nasal septum.
- The **OCCIPITAL** bone which forms the back of the skull

> **KEY NOTE** There are many openings present in the bones of the skull which act as passages for blood vessels and nerves entering and leaving the cranial cavity. For instance, there is a large opening at the base of the skull called the foramen magnum through which the spinal cord and blood vessels pass to and from the brain.

The Bones of the Face

There are fourteen facial bones in total and these are mainly in pairs, one on either side of the face:

TWO MAXILLAE – these are the largest bones of the face and they form the upper jaw and support the upper teeth. An important part of the maxillae are the maxillary sinuses which open into the nasal cavity.

ONE MANDIBLE – this is the only moveable bone of the skull and forms the lower jaw and supports the lower teeth

TWO ZYGOMATIC – these are the most prominent of the facial bones and they form the cheekbones.

TWO NASAL – these small bones form the bridge of the nose

TWO LACRIMAL – these are the smallest of the facial bones are located close to the medial part of the orbital cavity

TWO TURBINATE – these are layers of bone located either side of the outer walls of the nasal cavities

ONE VOMER – this is a single bone at the back of the nasal septum

TWO PALATINE – these are L-shaped bones which form the anterior part of the roof of the mouth

> **KEY NOTE** Indian Head Massage can help to make parts of the skeletal system such as the shoulders and neck more mobile by reducing restrictions in the joints, muscles and their fascia.

The Muscular System

There are over 600 skeletal or voluntary muscles in the body that collectively help to create body movement, stabilise joints and maintain body posture. Some skeletal muscles lie superficially, whilst those layered beneath them are known as deep muscles. Detailed below are the main muscles involved in Indian Head Massage.

MUSCLES IN THE REGION OF THE SHOULDERS, UPPER ARMS AND CHEST

Posterior Muscles

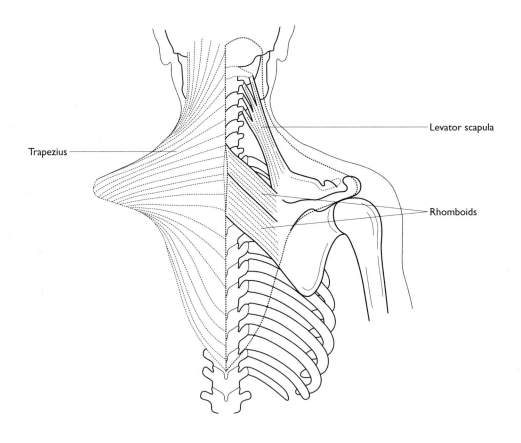

Trapezius

Levator scapula

Rhomboids

Name of Muscle	Position	Action	Key Note
TRAPEZIUS	a large triangular shaped muscle in the upper back that extends horizontally from the base of the skull and the cervical and thoracic vertebrae to the scapula. Its fibres are arranged in 3 groups: upper, middle and lower	the upper fibres raise the shoulder girdle; the middle fibres pull the scapula towards the vertebral column and the lower fibres draw the scapula and shoulder downward. When the trapezius is fixed in position by other muscles, it can pull the head backwards or to one side	this muscle tends to hold a lot of upper body tension, causing discomfort and restrictions in the neck and shoulder
LEVATOR SCAPULA	a straplike muscle that runs almost vertically through the neck, connecting the cervical vertebrae to the scapula	elevates and adducts the scapula	this muscle tends to become very tight, affecting mobility of the neck and shoulder
RHOMBOIDS	the fibres of these muscles lie between the scapulae, connecting them to the upper thoracic vertebrae	adduct the scapulae	these muscles are often very tight, resulting in aching and soreness in between the scapulae

Posterior Muscles cont.

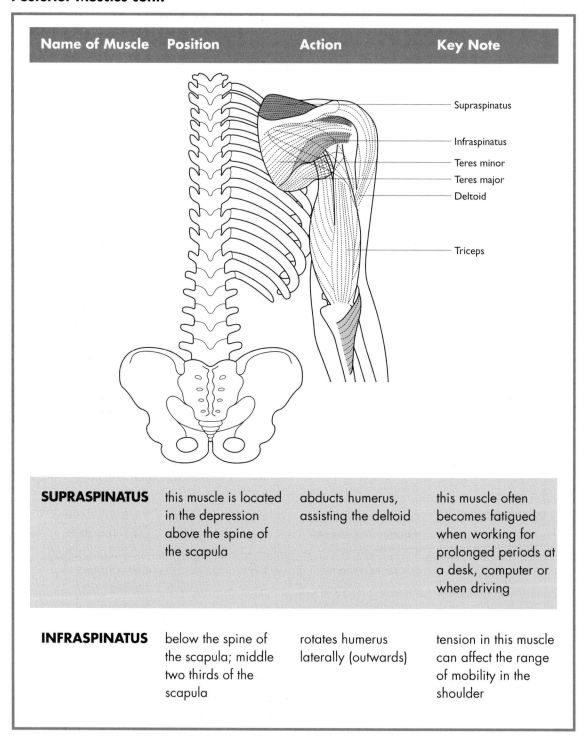

Name of Muscle	Position	Action	Key Note
			Supraspinatus
			Infraspinatus
			Teres minor
			Teres major
			Deltoid
			Triceps
SUPRASPINATUS	this muscle is located in the depression above the spine of the scapula	abducts humerus, assisting the deltoid	this muscle often becomes fatigued when working for prolonged periods at a desk, computer or when driving
INFRASPINATUS	below the spine of the scapula; middle two thirds of the scapula	rotates humerus laterally (outwards)	tension in this muscle can affect the range of mobility in the shoulder

Posterior Muscles cont.

Name of Muscle	Position	Action	Key Note
TERES MAJOR	across the bottom lateral edge of the scapula	adducts and medially (inwardly) rotates humerus	tension in this muscle restricts the mobility of the shoulder and upper arm
TERES MINOR	across the lateral edge of the scapula, above teres major	rotates humerus laterally (outwards)	tension in this muscle restricts the mobility of the shoulder and upper arm
TRICEPS	posterior of the humerus	extension of the forearm	this muscle becomes tight when the body assumes a tension posture (hunched shoulders and arms and elbows hugged tight against the body.)

Anterior

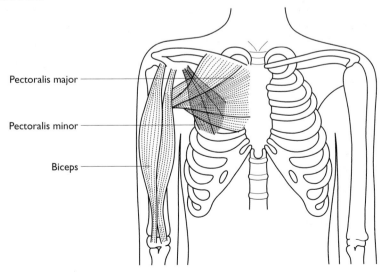

Pectoralis major

Pectoralis minor

Biceps

Name of Muscle	Position	Action	Key Note
PECTORALIS MINOR	a thin flat muscle that lies beneath pectoralis major	draws the shoulder downwards and forwards	tightness in this muscle may cause construction of the chest or postural distortions (such as rounded shoulders)
SERRATUS ANTERIOR	a broad curved shaped muscle located on the side of the chest, across the sides of the rib cage below the axilla	draws the scapula forwards and pops it upwards. It is used when pushing	this muscle can be affected by chest and breathing difficulties
PECTORALIS MAJOR	a thick fan-shaped muscle, covering the anterior surface of the upper chest. Its fibres extend from the centre of the thorax out to the humerus	adducts arm, medially (inwardly) pops arm	tightness in this muscle may cause construction of the chest or postural distortions (such as rounded shoulders)
DELTOID	a thick triangular muscle that caps the top of the humerus and shoulder	abducts arm, draws the arm backwards and forwards	this muscle tends to hold upper body tension
BICEPS	anterior of the upper arm	flexion of the forearm	this muscle becomes tight when the body assumes a tension posture (hunched shoulders and arms and elbows hugged tight against the body).

Muscles Located in the Region of the Neck

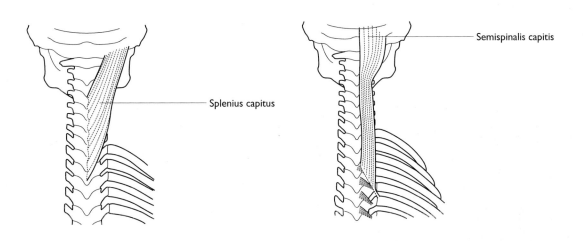

Splenius capitus

Semispinalis capitis

Name of Muscle	Position	Action	Key Note
STERNOMASTOID	this is a long muscle in the side of the neck that extends upwards from the sternum to the mastoid process behind the ear	together they flex the neck. Individually they turn the head to the opposite side	this muscle is used when nodding and becomes very tense when the head is consistently turned to one side, or pointing downwards, as in working on the telephone and at a desk
PLATYSMA	a thin sheet-like muscle; its fibres extend from the chest up the sides of the neck to the chin	depresses the mandible and lower lip	this muscle is used when yawning and when pouting

Muscles Located in the Region of the Neck cont.

Name of Muscle	Position	Action	Key Note
SPLENIUS CAPITUS	this is a broad strap-like muscle located in the back of the neck. It connects the base of the skull to the vertebrae in the neck and upper thorax	acting together these muscles bring the head into an upright position	these muscles become over contracted when the neck is thrust forwards and downwards, as in working at a desk. They also become tight when turning the head to one side to hold the ear to the receiver of the telephone
SEMISPINALIS CAPITIS	this is a broad sheet-like muscle extending upwards from the vertebrae in the neck and thorax to the occipital bone	extends the head, bends it to one side, or rotates it	see above
LONGISSIMUS CAPITIS	a narrow band of muscle that ascends from the vertebrae of the neck and thorax to the temporal bone of the skull	extends the head, bends it to one side, or rotates it.	see above

Muscles located in the Region of the Head

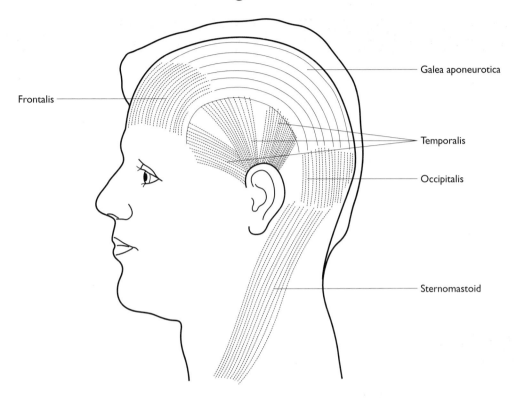

Galea aponeurotica

Frontalis

Temporalis

Occipitalis

Sternomastoid

Name of Muscle	Position	Action	Key Note
OCCIPITALIS	extends over the back of the skull	moves the scalp backwards	this muscle is united to the frontalis muscle by a broad tendon called the epicranial aponeurosis which covers the skull like a cap
FRONTALIS	extends over the front of the skull	moves the scalp forwards, raises the eyebrows and wrinkles the forehead	see Occipitalis

Muscles located in the Region of the Neck cont.

Name of Muscle	Position	Action	Key Note
TEMPORALIS	a fan-shaped muscle on the side of the skull above and in front of the ear	elevates and retracts the lower jaw	this muscle become over-tight and painful in the condition known as Temporomandibular joint dysfunction syndrome.

Muscles in the Region of the Face

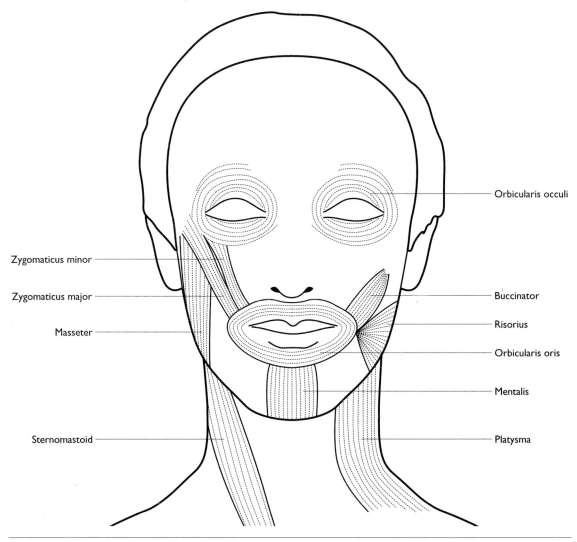

Name of Muscle	Position	Action	Key Note
ORBICULARIS OCCULI	a ringlike band of muscle (called a sphincter muscle) that surrounds the eye. It lies in the subcutaneous tissue of the eyelid	closes the eye	this muscle is used when blinking or winking. It also compresses the lacrimal gland aiding the flow of tears
ORBICULARIS ORIS	a ringlike band of muscle that encircles the mouth.	closes the lips	this muscle is used when shaping the lips for speech and when kissing. Its also contracts when tense, as the lips tend to tighten
ZYGOMATICUS	this muscle extends from the zygomatic arch downwards to the corner of the mouth	raises the corner of the mouth	this muscle is used when smiling or laughing
RISORIUS	a triangular shaped muscle that lies horizontally on the cheek, joining at the corners of the mouth	draws corners of the mouth laterally	this muscle is used when grinning
BUCCINATOR	this muscle is located in the wall of the cheek; its fibres are directed forward from the bones of the jaws to the angle of the mouth	this muscle helps hold food in contact with the teeth when chewing and compresses the cheek	this muscle is located in the wall of the cheek where tension in the face can accumulate. This muscle is also used when blowing

Muscles in the Region of the Face cont.

Name of Muscle	Position	Action	Key Note
MENTALIS	radiates from the lower lip over the centre of the chin	elevates the lower lip and wrinkles the chin	this muscle is used when expressing displeasure and when pouting
MASSETER	a thick flattened muscle whose fibres extend downwards from the zygomatic arch to the mandible	raises the lower jaw; is a muscle of mastication	this muscle holds a lot of tension and can be felt just in front of the ear when the teeth are clenched.

KEY NOTE Muscular tension is often a sign of emotional as well as physical stress. Indian Head Massage can help to relieve pain from tight, sore muscles as well as relieve muscular fatigue, by increasing blood flow which increases the amount of oxygen and nutrition into the muscles and encourages elimination of waste, absorbing the products of fatigue.

THE BLOOD FLOW TO THE HEAD AND NECK

The circulatory system comprises of blood, the heart and the vast network of circulatory vessels known as arteries, veins and capillaries. The primary function of the circulatory system is transportation. Within the cardiovascular system there are two circuits: the pulmonary circulation and the systemic circulation.

The pulmonary circulation brings deoxygenated blood from the right ventricle of the heart to the alveoli of the lungs to release carbon dioxide and to regain oxygen. Oxygenated blood returns to the left atrium of the heart and moves into the systemic circuit with the contraction of the left ventricle. The systemic circuit carries oxygenated blood around the body via the body's main artery: the aorta.

On leaving the left ventricle the aorta emerges from the top of the heart. It passes superiorly for a short distance as the ascending aorta and curves to form the arch of the aorta before it passes inferiorly as the descending aorta. As the aorta emerges from the heart it subdivides to form the main trunk called the **BRACHIOCEPHALIC TRUNK** which splits and forms the **COMMON CAROTID ARTERY** which supplies oxygenated blood to the head, face and neck and the **SUBCLAVIAN ARTERY**, which supplies blood to the shoulders, chest wall, arms, back and central nervous system.

ARTERIAL BLOOD SUPPLY TO THE HEAD AND NECK

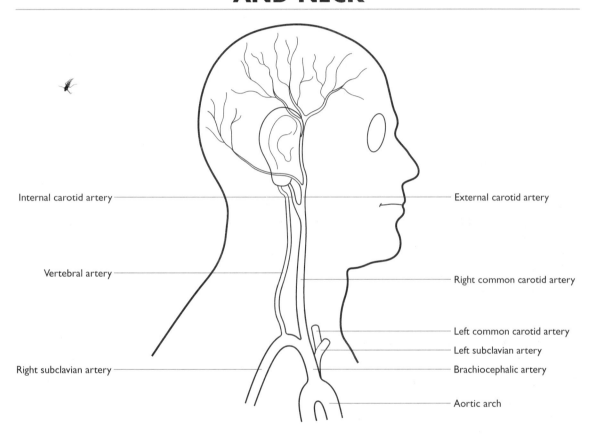

Internal carotid artery

External carotid artery

Vertebral artery

Right common carotid artery

Left common carotid artery

Left subclavian artery

Right subclavian artery

Brachiocephalic artery

Aortic arch

Blood is supplied to parts within the neck, head and brain through branches of the subclavian and common carotid arteries.

The **COMMON CAROTID ARTERY** extends from the brachiocephalic trunk and extends on each side of the neck and divides at the level of the larynx into two branches: the internal carotid artery and the **EXTERNAL CAROTID ARTERY**.

The **INTERNAL CAROTID ARTERY** passes through the temporal bone of the skull to supply oxygenated blood to the brain, eyes, forehead and part of the nose.

The **EXTERNAL CAROTID ARTERY** is divided into branches (facial, temporal and occipital arteries) which supply the skin and muscles of the face, side and back of the head respectively. This vessel also supplies more superficial structures of the head and neck; these include the salivary glands, scalp, teeth, nose, throat, tongue and thyroid gland.

The **VERTEBRAL ARTERIES** are a main division of the subclavian artery. They arise from the subclavian arteries in the base of the neck near the tip of the lungs. They pass upwards through the openings (foramina) of transverse processes of the cervical vertebrae and unite to form a single basilar artery. The basilar artery then terminates by dividing into two posterior cerebral arteries that supply the occipital and temporal lobes of the cerebrum.

VENOUS DRAINAGE FROM THE HEAD AND NECK

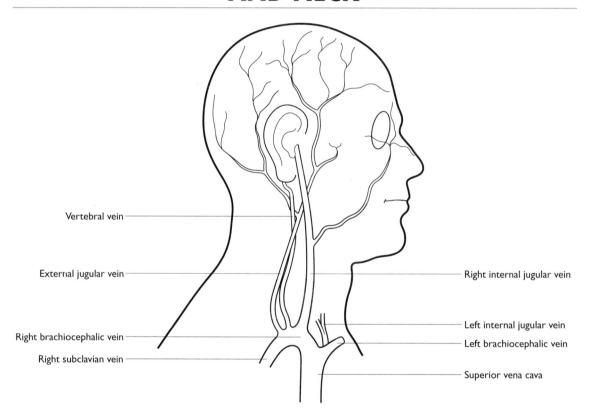

The majority of blood draining from the head is passed into three pairs of veins: the external jugular veins, the internal jugular veins and the vertebral veins. Within the brain all veins lead to the internal jugular veins.

The **EXTERNAL JUGULAR VEIN** is smaller than the internal jugular and lies superficial to it. It receives blood from superficial regions of the face, scalp and neck. The external jugular veins descend on either side of the neck, passing over the sternomastoid muscles and beneath the platysma. They empty into the right and left subclavian veins in the base of the neck.

The **INTERNAL JUGULAR VEIN** forms the major venous drainage of the head and neck and is a deep vein that parallels the common carotid artery. They collect deoxygenated blood from the brain and pass downwards through the neck besides the common carotid arteries and join the subclavian veins.

The **VERTEBRAL VEINS** descend from the transverse openings (or foramina) of the cervical vertebrae and enter the subclavian veins. The vertebral veins drain deep structures of the neck such as the vertebrae and muscles.

> **KEY NOTE** Indian Head Massage can help to enhance the circulation of blood and hence increase cell nutrition and elimination of cellular waste to and from the head and neck. The improved circulation to head also helps to refresh the brain, helping to relieve stress, tension and fatigue.

The Lymphatic System

The lymphatic system is a one-way drainage system in that it removes excess fluid from the body's tissues and returns it to the circulatory system. It is also important in helping the body to fight infection.

Lymphatic vessels form a network of tubes that extend all over the body. The smallest of the vessels – lymphatic capillaries, end blindly in the body's tissues. Here they collect a liquid called lymph which leaks out of the body capillaries and accumulates in the tissues. Once collected, lymph flows in one direction along progressively larger lymph vessels. Along the network of lymph vessels are lymph nodes which filter bacteria and micro-organisms from the lymph as it passes through them. The cleansed lymph is then collected by two main lymphatic ducts (the thoracic and the right lymphatic ducts) which empty the lymph into the bloodstream.

The lymphatic system therefore returns the excess fluid which accumulates in the body's tissues back into the bloodstream, whilst at the same time filters micro-organisms and releases antibodies to help the body to fight infection.

> **KEY NOTE** The movement of lymph throughout the lymphatic system is known as lymphatic drainage and it begins in the lymph capillaries. The movement of lymph out of the tissue spaces and into the lymph capillaries, is assisted by the pressure exerted by the compression of skeletal muscles. This explains why techniques such as Indian Head massage are an effective way of draining lymph.

LYMPHATIC DRAINAGE OF THE HEAD AND NECK

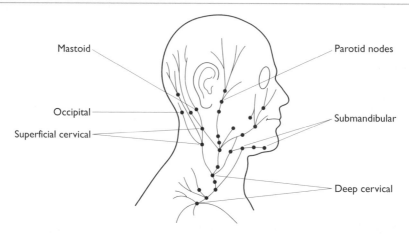

There main groups of lymph nodes relating to the head and neck

Name of Lymph Nodes	Position	Areas lymph is drained from
CERVICAL (DEEP)	deep within the neck, located along the path of the larger blood vessels (carotid artery and internal jugular vein)	drains lymph from the larynx, oesophagus, posterior of the scalp and neck, superficial part of chest and arm
CERVICAL (SUPERFICIAL)	located at the side of the neck, over the sternomastoid muscle	drains lymph from the lower part of the ear and the cheek region
SUBMANDIBULAR	beneath the mandible	drains chin, lips, nose, cheeks and tongue
OCCIPITAL	at the base of the skull	drains back of scalp, and the upper part of neck
MASTOID (POST AURICULAR)	behind the ear in the region of the mastoid process	drains the skin of the ear and the temporal region of the scalp
PAROTID	at the angle of the jaw	drains nose, eyelids and ear.

The right side of the head, neck and right arm drains into the right lymphatic duct and then into the right subclavian vein. The left side of the head, neck, the left arm, (as well as the lower limbs and abdomen) drain into the left subclavian vein.

The Nervous System

The nervous system comprises of the brain, spinal cord and nerves which together form communication networks to co-ordinate the various actions of the body. The nervous system contains billions of interconnecting neurones which are designed to transmit nerve impulses. There are three types of neurones:

SENSORY NEURONES: these receive stimuli from sensory organs and receptors and transmit the impulse to the spinal cord and brain. Sensations transmitted by sensory neurones include heat, cold, pain, taste, smell, sight and hearing.

MOTOR NEURONES: these conduct impulses away from the brain and the spinal cord to muscles and glands to stimulate them into carrying out their activities.

ASSOCIATION (MIXED) NEURONES: these link sensory and motor neurones, helping to form the complex pathways that enable the brain to interpret incoming sensory messages, decide on what should be done and send out instructions in response along motor pathways to keep the body functioning properly.

The nervous system has two main parts which both possess unique structural and functional characteristics.

- **THE CENTRAL NERVOUS SYSTEM** (the main control system) that consist of the **BRAIN** and the **SPINAL CORD**
- **THE PERIPHERAL NERVOUS SYSTEM** consisting of 31 pairs of **SPINAL NERVES**, 12 pairs of **CRANIAL NERVES** and the **AUTONOMIC NERVOUS SYSTEM**

THE CENTRAL NERVOUS SYSTEM

The central nervous system, consisting of the brain and spinal cord, is covered by a special type of connective tissue called the meninges. The meninges has three layers:

- the **DURA MATER**, which is the outer protective fibrous connective tissue sheath covering the brain and spinal cord
- the **PIA MATER**, the innermost later, is attached to the surface of organs and is richly supplied with blood vessels to nourish the underlying tissues
- the **ARACHNOID MATER** which provides a space for the blood vessels and circulation of cerebrospinal fluid

Cerebrospinal fluid is a clear fluid derived from the blood and secreted into the inner cavities of the brain. It carries some nutrients to the nerve tissue and carries waste away, but its main function is to protect the central nervous system by acting as a shock absorber for the delicate nervous tissue.

THE BRAIN

The brain is an extremely complex mass of nervous tissue lying within the skull. It is the main communication centre of the nervous system and its function is to co-ordinate the nerve stimuli received and effect the correct responses.

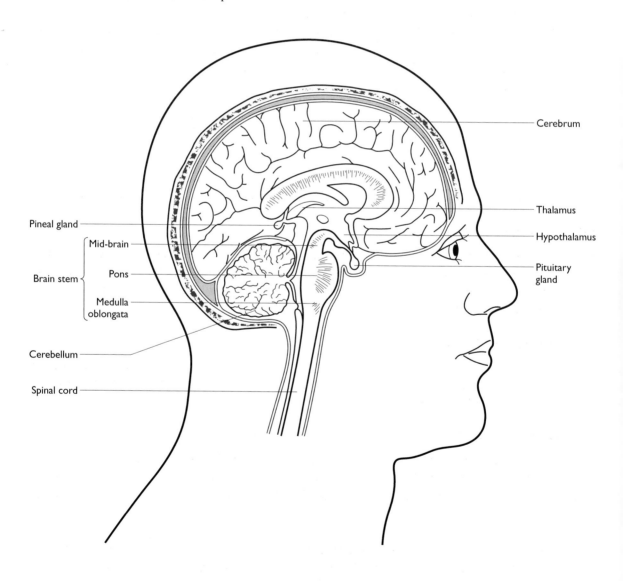

The main parts of the brain include the following:

THE CEREBRUM – this is the largest portion of the brain and makes up the front and top part of the brain. It is divided into two large cerebral hemispheres. The outer layer of the cerebrum is called the cerebral cortex and is the region where the main functions of the cerebrum are carried out. The cortex is concerned with all forms of conscious activity: sensations such as vision, touch, hearing, taste and smell; control of voluntary movements; reasoning; emotion; and memory.

The cortex of each cerebral hemisphere has a number of functional areas:

- **SENSORY AREAS** – these receive impulses from sensory organs all over the body; there are separate sensory areas for vision, hearing, touch, taste and smell
- **MOTOR AREAS** – these areas have motor connections through motor nerve fibres with voluntary muscles all over the body
- **ASSOCIATION AREAS** – in these areas association takes place between information from the sensory areas and remembered information from past experiences. Conscious thought then takes place and decisions are made which often result in conscious motor activity controlled by motor areas.

The brain requires a continuous supply of glucose and oxygen as it is unable to store glycogen, unlike the liver and muscles.

The Thalamus

This is a relay and interpretation centre for all sensory impulses, except olfaction (sense of smell).

The Hypothalamus

This is a small structure that governs many important homeostatic functions. It regulates the autonomic nervous system and endocrine system by governing the pituitary gland. It controls hunger, thirst, temperature regulation, anger, aggression, hormones, sexual behaviour, sleep patterns and consciousness.

The Pituitary Gland

This is a pea-shaped body attached beneath the hypothalamus in a bony cavity at the base of the skull. It is known as the master endocrine gland as its hormones control and stimulate other glands to produce their hormones.

The Pineal Gland

This is a pea-sized mass of nerve tissue attached by a stalk in the central part of the brain. It is located deep between the cerebral hemispheres, where it is attached to the upper portion of the thalamus. The pineal gland secretes a hormone called melatonin, which it synthesises from serotonin.

The pineal gland is involved in the regulation of circadian rhythms, patterns of repeated activity that are associated with the environmental cycles of day and night such as sleep/wake rhythms. The pineal gland is also thought to influence the mood.

The Cerebellum

The cerebellum is a cauliflower-shaped structure located at the posterior of the cranium, below the cerebrum. The cerebellum is concerned with muscle tone, the co-ordination of skeletal muscles and balance.

The Brain Stem contains 3 main structures:

- **THE MID-BRAIN** – this contains the main nerve pathways connecting the cerebrum and the lower nervous system, as well as certain visual and auditory reflexes that co-ordinate head and eye movements with things seen and heard.
- **THE PONS** – this is below the mid-brain and relays messages from the cerebral cortex to the spinal cord
- **THE MEDULLA OBLONGATA** – this is often considered the most vital part of the brain. It is an enlarged continuation of the spinal cord and connects the brain with the spinal cord. Control centres within the medulla oblongata include for those for the heart, lungs and intestines.

THE SPINAL CORD – an extension of the brain stem which extends from an opening at the base of the skull down to the second lumbar vertebra. Its function is to relay impulses to and from the brain.

THE PERIPHERAL NERVOUS SYSTEM which consists of cable-like nerves that link the central nervous system to the rest of the body.

It consists of:

THIRTY-ONE PAIRS OF SPINAL NERVES – these nerves pass out of the spinal cord and each has two thin branches which link it with the autonomic nervous system. Spinal nerves receive sensory impulses from the body and transmit motor signals to specific regions of the body, thereby providing two-way communication between the central nervous system and the body.

Each of the spinal nerves are numbered and are named according to the level of the spinal column from which they emerge. There are:

- eight cervical
- twelve thoracic
- five lumbar
- five sacral
- one coccygeal

Each spinal nerve is divided into several branches, forming a network of nerves or plexuses which supply different parts of the body:

THE CERVICAL PLEXUSES of the neck supply the skin and muscles of the head, neck, and upper region of the shoulders

THE BRACHIAL PLEXUSES supply the skin and muscles of the arm, shoulder and upper chest

THE LUMBAR PLEXUSES supply the front and sides of the abdominal wall and part of the thigh

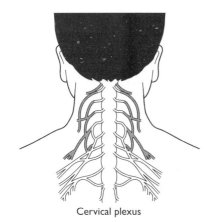

Cervical plexus

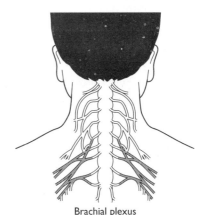

Brachial plexus

THE SACRAL PLEXUSES at the base of the abdomen supply the skin and muscles and organs of the pelvis

THE COCCYGEAL PLEXUS supplies the skin in the area of the coccyx and the muscles of the pelvic floor

TWELVE PAIRS OF CRANIAL NERVES – these nerves connect directly to the brain and between them they provide a nerve supply to sensory organs, muscles and skin of the head and neck.

Some of the nerves are mixed, containing both motor and sensory nerves, while others are either sensory or motor.

I OLFACTORY NERVE
This is a sensory nerve of olfaction (smell)

II OPTIC NERVE
This is a sensory nerve of vision

III OCULOMOTOR NERVE
This is a mixed nerve that innervates both internal and external muscles of the eye and a muscle of the upper eyelid

IV TROCHLEAR NERVE
This is the smallest of the cranial nerves and is a motor nerve that innervates the superior oblique muscle of the eyeball that helps you look upwards

V TRIGEMENAL NERVE

This is a mixed nerve (containing motor and sensory nerves) that conducts impulses to and from several areas in the face and neck. It also controls the muscles of mastication (the masseter, the temporalis and the pterygoids). It has 3 main branches – ophthalmic branch, maxillary branch and mandibular branch.

THE OPHTHALMIC BRANCH carries sensations from the eye, nasal cavity, skin of forehead, upper eyelid, eyebrow and part of the nose

THE MAXILLARY BRANCH carries sensations from the lower eyelid, upper lip, gums, teeth, cheek, nose, palate and part of the pharynx

THE MANDIBULAR BRANCH carries sensations from the lower gums, teeth, lips, palate and part of the tongue

VI ABDUCENS

This is a mixed nerve that innervates only the lateral rectus muscle of the eye, which helps you look to the side

VII FACIAL

This is a mixed nerve that conducts impulses to and from several areas in the face and neck. The sensory branches are associated with the taste receptors on the tongue and the motor fibres transmit impulses to the muscles of facial expression

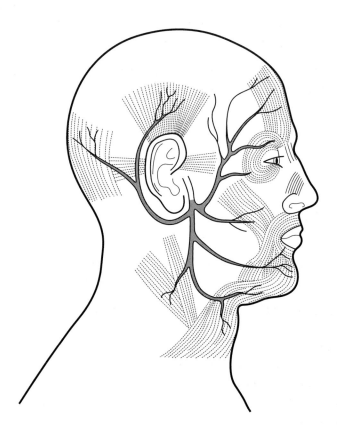

VIII VESTIBULOCOCHLEAR
This is a sensory nerve that transmits impulses generated by auditory stimuli and stimuli related to equilibrium, balance and movement

IX GLOSSOPHARYNGEAL
This is a mixed nerve that innervates structures in the mouth and throat. It supplies motor fibres to part of the pharynx and to the parotid salivary glands and sensory fibres to the posterior third of the tongue and the soft palate

X VAGUS
This is unlike the other cranial nerves in that it has branches to numerous organs in the thorax and abdomen as well as the neck. It supplies motor nerve fibres to the muscles of swallowing and motor nerve fibres to the heart and organs of the chest cavity. Sensory fibres carry impulses from the organs of the abdominal cavity and the sensation of taste from the mouth

XI ACCESSORY
This functions primarily as a motor nerve, innervating muscles in the neck and upper back (such as the trapezius and the sternomastoid), as well as muscles of the palate, pharynx and larynx

XII HYPOGLOSSAL
This is a motor nerve that innervates the muscles of the tongue.

THE AUTONOMIC NERVOUS SYSTEM – the part of the nervous system that control the automatic body activities of smooth and cardiac muscle and the activities of glands. It is divided into the sympathetic and parasympathetic divisions, which possess complementary responses.

The activity of the sympathetic system is to prepare the body for expending energy and dealing with emergency situations. Its effects include:
- increased heartbeat
- increased respiration rate
- dilation of skeletal blood vessels
- stimulation of the adrenal and sweat glands
- increased conversion of glycogen to glucose by liver
- pupils dilation
- inhibited salivation
- decreased gastrointestinal activity

The parasympathetic nervous system balances the action of the sympathetic division by working to converse energy and create the conditions needed for rest and sleep.

Effects of the **PARASYMPATHETIC ACTIVITY** include:
- resting heart rate
- resting respiratory rate
- constriction of skeletal blood vessels
- increased gastro-intestinal activity
- pupil construction
- stimulated salivation

KEY NOTE The sympathetic nervous system is activated at time of anger, fright, anxiety or any type of emotional upset, whether real or imagined. Indian Head Massage can help to decrease the effects of the sympathetic nervous system and hence reduce stress levels. It also helps to activate the parasympathetic nervous system, thus promoting relaxation and creating the conditions needed for rest and sleep. It can also help to reduce stress hormones such as cortisol by activating the relaxation process. Indian Head Massage is also thought to increase serotonin levels which can help to decrease stress levels and depression.

RESPIRATION

Oxygen is needed by every cell of the body for survival and delivery ; respiration is the process by which the living cells of the body receive a constant supply of oxygen and remove carbon dioxide and other gases.

The respiratory system consists of the nose, the pharynx, the larynx, the trachea, the bronchi and the lungs which provide the passageway for air in and out of the body.

During inhalation air is drawn in through the nose, pharynx, trachea and bronchi and into the lungs. Inside the lungs each bronchus divides to form a tree of tubes called bronchioles which progressively increase in diameter and end in microscopic air sacs called alveoli. Oxygen from the air that reaches the alveoli diffuses through the alveolar walls and into the surrounding blood capillaries. This oxygen-rich blood is carried first to the heart and is then pumped to cells throughout the body. Carbon dioxide diffuses out of the blood into the alveoli and is removed from the body during exhalation.

The Mechanism of Respiration

The mechanism of respiration is the means by which air is drawn in and out of the lungs and is an active process where the muscles of respiration contract to increase the volume of the thoracic cavity.

The major muscle of respiration is the diaphragm. During inspiration the diaphragm contracts and flattens, increasing the volume of the thoracic cavity and is responsible for 75% of air movement into the lungs. The external intercostals are also involved in respiration and upon contraction they increase the depth of the thoracic cavity by pulling the ribs upwards and outwards.

The external intercostal muscles are responsible for bringing approximately 25% of the volume of air into the lungs. The combined contraction of the diaphragm and the external inter-costals increase the thoracic cavity, which then decreases the pressure inside the thorax so that

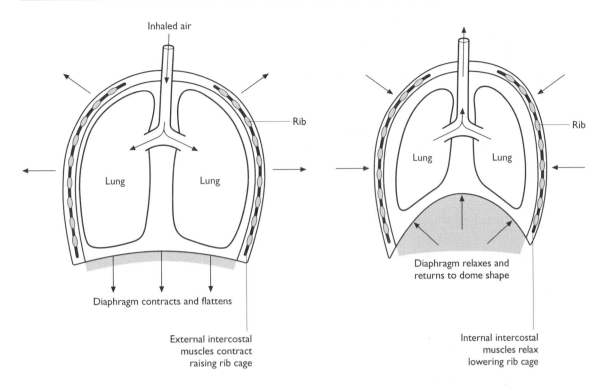

Inhaled air

Rib

Lung   Lung

Diaphragm contracts and flattens

External intercostal
muscles contract
raising rib cage

Lung   Lung

Rib

Diaphragm relaxes and
returns to dome shape

Internal intercostal
muscles relax
lowering rib cage

air from outside of the body enters the lungs. Other accessory muscles which assist in inspiration include the sternomastoid, serratus anterior, pectoralis minor, pectoralis major and the scalene muscles in the neck.

During normal respiration the process of expiration is passive and is brought about by the relaxation of the diaphragm and the external intercostal muscles. This increases the internal pressure inside the thorax so that air is pushed out of the lungs.

In forced expiration, the process of expiration becomes active and is assisted by muscles such as the internal intercostals which help to depress the ribs. Abdominal muscles such as the external and internal obliques, rectus abdominus and the transversus abdominus help to compress the abdomen and the force the diaphragm upwards, thus assisting expiration.

> **KEY NOTE** Breathing affects both our physiological and psychological state. By freeing tight respiratory muscles, Indian Head Massage can help to increase the vital capacity and function of the lungs.

Self Assessment Questions

1. a) Name the 5 layers of the epidermis

   b) Explain the process of cell regeneration in the skin

2. Where does hair growth originate from?

3. Explain 3 factors that affect hair growth

4. State four functions of the skin

5. Name the bones of the shoulder girdle

6. What are the bones of the neck called and how many are there?

7. Name the following bones of the skull

a) the bones that form the sides of the skull above and around the ears

b) The bone that forms the anterior part of the skull

c) The bone at the base of the skull

d) The bones that form the upper sides of the skull and the back of the roof of the skull

8. Name the following bones of the face

a) the bone that forms the lower jaw

b) the bones that form the cheekbones

c) the bones that form the upper jaw and support the upper teeth

9. In each of the following, i) Identify the name of the muscle; ii) State its action.

a) This muscle extends from the chest up the sides of the neck to the chin

b) This is a long muscle which extends from the sternum to the mastoid process behind the ear

c) A fan shaped muscle on the side of the skull above and in front of the ear

d) This broad sheet-like muscle extends over the front of the skull

e) A ringlike band of muscle that surrounds the eye

f) This muscle is located in the wall of the cheek

g) This muscle extends from the lower lip over the centre of the chin

h) A triangular-shaped muscle that lies horizontally on the cheek, joining at the corners of the mouth

10. Name the blood vessels that are responsible for supplying oxygenated blood to the head and neck

11. Name the blood vessels responsible for draining deoxygenated blood from the head and neck

12. Identify the following lymph nodes

a) drain lymph from the back of the scalp and the upper part of the neck

b) located at the side of the neck over the sternomastoid muscle

c) located beneath the mandible

d) drain the skin of the ear and the temporal region of the scalp

e) drain lymph from the larynx, oesophagus, posterior of the scalp and neck, superficial part of the chest and arm

13. Name the two main parts of the nervous system

14. State the functional significance of the following parts of the brain

a) the cerebrum

b) the cerebellum

c) the medulla oblongata

15. Name the parts of the peripheral nervous system

16. Name the facial nerve that has 3 main branches and conduct impulses to and from several areas in the face and neck

17. Describe the effects of the following

a) sympathetic nervous system

b) parasympathetic nervous system

18. Describe the mechanism of respiration

CHAPTER 3

Consultation for Indian Head Massage

A client consultation involves professional communication between a client and a therapist and is a critical skill that helps establish a positive and trusting therapeutic relationship between both parties. The time spent in establishing a professional relationship with the client will often result in client satisfaction and their continued patronage. Therapists therefore need to have effective communication skills which involve both talking and listening to clients in order to be able record and respond positively to the information elicited.

At end of this chapter you will be able to:

- Carry out a consultation for Indian Head Massage
- Understand how contra-indications and precautions may affect the proposed treatment
- Liaise with other health care professionals
- Formulate a treatment plan for Indian Head Massage

Client Consultation Skills

As with all holistic therapy treatments, a consultation for Indian Head Massage involves one-to-one communication. During a consultation, a therapist's contact with the client involves talking, listening, non-verbal communication, as well as the recording of written information. When carrying out a consultation, therapists need to adopt a warm, calm, open and understanding attitude towards the client, in order to facilitate a channel of positive communication.

Clients presenting for treatment may be nervous or apprehensive about the treatment and it is therefore important for a therapist to adopt a sensitive, respectful and friendly attitude to the client at all times. Although talking is an important part of a consultation, one of the most critical skills a therapist can develop is in listening. Through effective listening, a therapist can customise the treatment with the aim of meeting the client's needs and expectations. It is important for therapists to realise that clients often communicate without the spoken word and non-verbal messages may be projected without the client's awareness. Therapists therefore need to be aware of what a client may be communicating in the tone of their words, gestures they may make, the posture they may present or by their facial expressions. With this in mind, therapists may realise that there may be a difference between what a client is expressing in words and what their body language may be indicating.

Consultation Environment

In order to facilitate a positive approach to a consultation, it is important to be aware of the environment in which it is undertaken. The environment for a consultation should ideally be private in order to respect the client's privacy and dignity in disclosing personal information. Attention to aspects such as lighting, smell, temperature and comfort of a consultation area can all help to aid client relaxation and decrease apprehension.

Client Education

Consultations provide an ideal opportunity for therapists to educate clients on what Indian Head Massage involves, its potential benefits along with the costs and time involved. Clients do not usually want to become passive recipients of the treatment and if they are to invest time and money in a therapy they need to be educated so that they become partners in their healing process. Consultations also provide the client with the opportunity to ask questions about the treatment for reassurance and clarification.

Based on the information and the education provided about the service, the client is then responsible for making a decision as to the treatment objectives. It is the therapist's responsibility to provide a treatment to suit their needs but to accurately inform them if their objectives and expectations are unrealistic. It is essential for therapists to stress to clients the importance of regular treatments to maintain long term benefits.

Clients may also be empowered to take charge of their own healing through client education of adjustments to lifestyle, posture and the correct use of ergonomics (the positioning of furniture at work).

Client Confidentiality

Client confidentiality is an important factor in a therapeutic relationship between a client and a therapist. Clients should be reassured that all information recorded will remain confidential and is stored securely, and that no information will be disclosed to a third party without the client's written consent. Maintaining client confidentiality will also help to establish a trusting professional relationship between a client and a therapist.

Written Documentation

Written documentation is essential in a consultation as it provides a systematic and continued record of the client's progress. Consultation documents should always be used as a guide to facilitate communication, and questions may need to be phrased in a certain way to maximise communication and receive qualitative information. For instance, upon asking a client about their stress levels, they may merely reply "high". In order to gain more information, a therapist may pose the question "in which part of the body do you feel stress most often?" or "what factors are involved in your stress levels being high at the moment?"

It is important for therapists to realise that information received from the client is largely subjective in that it is from their viewpoint, and this information may differ from what is evaluated by the therapist.

Important information to be discussed during the consultation are any factors which may affect their physical and emotional health such as medical history, diet, lifestyle, occupation, sleep patterns, exercise and relaxation which may all contribute to an overall picture of the client from a holistic point if view. Besides talking, listening and recording informed on a client's records, client consultation involves other assessment skills such as:

- **VISUAL ASSESSMENT** – this commences from the first point of contact with the client. Observations as to the client's mood, rate and depth of breathing, posture and gait may all help to contribute to the state of the client's physical and emotional health.
- **MANUAL ASSESSMENT OF THE TISSUES** – the most effective form of communication a therapist can facilitate is in touch, and throughout the Indian Head Massage treatment the therapist can assess the tissues for tension, restrictions, temperature changes etc.

CONTRA-INDICATIONS AND CAUTIONS

Despite Indian Head Massage being an extremely safe and effective treatment, it is important for therapists to be aware of:

1. Conditions that are contra-indicated and for which treatment cannot be provided
2. Conditions that may require referral to the client's GP or another professional before treatment may be given
3. Conditions that may present certain restrictions and for which treatment may need to be adapted
4. Special factors which may influence the treatment length or techniques applied

Knowledge of contra-indications and precautions enables a therapist to work safely and effectively. Here are some examples:

- **HIGH TEMPERATURE OR FEVER** – is a contra-indication because of the risk of spreading infection as a result of the increased circulation

- **ACUTE INFECTIOUS DISEASE** – these would be contra-indicated due to the fact that the condition would be highly contagious
- **SKIN OR SCALP INFECTIONS** – these may be worsened and spread by the massage.

COMMON SKIN INFECTIONS

HERPES SIMPLEX – this condition is normally found on the face and around the lips. It begins as an itching sensation, followed by erythema and a group of small blisters which then weep and form crusts. The condition normally persists for approximately two to three weeks but will reappear at times of stress, ill health or exposure to sunlight.

IMPETIGO – this is a superficial contagious inflammatory disease caused by streptococcal and staphylococcal bacteria. It is commonly seen on the face and around the ears, and features include weeping blisters which dry to form honey coloured crusts.

RINGWORM – this is a fungal infection of the skin, which begins as small red papules that gradually increase in size to form a ring. Itching is pronounced with this condition and lesions may be found all over the body.

SCABIES – this is a contagious parasitic condition, caused by the female mite who burrows into the horny layer of the skin where she lays her eggs. The first noticeable signs of this condition is severe itching and small reddish vesicles in the affected areas.

EYE INFECTION

CONJUNCTIVITIS is when the conjunctiva of the eye becomes inflamed and becomes red and swollen, producing a water or pus-containing discharge. Conjunctivitis may be caused by infection by bacteria or viruses (in which case it usually spreads rapidly to the other eye), or may be caused by physical or chemical irritation.

COMMON SCALP INFECTIONS

FOLLICULITIS is a bacterial infection of the hair follicles of the skin and appears as a small pustule at the base of a hair follicle. There is redness, swelling and pain around the hair follicle.

PEDICULOSIS (LICE) is an infestation (wingless insect) that feeds on human and animal blood. With head lice nits may be found in the hair. Nits are pearl-grey or brown, oval structures found on the hair shaft close to the scalp. The scalp may appear red and raw due to scratching. A client affected by body lice will complain of itching especially in the shoulder, back and buttock area.

TINEA CAPITIS is a fungal infection of the scalp (Ringworm) and appears as painless, round, hairless patches on the scalp. Itching may be present and the lesion may appear red and scaly.

It is important for therapists to avoid all contact with lesions, and clients with any skin or scalp infection should be advised to seek advice and treatment from their GP.

- **RECENT HAEMORRHAGE** – haemorrhaging is excessive bleeding which may be either external or internal. Massage should be avoided due to the risk of blood spillage from blood vessels.
INTOXICATION – it is inadvisable to carry out treatment whilst a client is under the influence of alcohol as the increase of blood flow to the head could make them feel dizzy and nauseous.
- **RECENT HEAD OR NECK INJURY** – in the case of a recent blow to the head with concussion, or an acute neck injury due to a recent accident, such as whiplash, it would be inadvisable to treat due to the risk of exacerbating the condition and increasing the inflammation and pain. However, if there is an old injury, massage may help to reduce scar tissue, decrease pain and increase mobility. Always obtain medical clearance to ensure the client's condition is suitable for treatment.
- **RECENT SURGERY** – depending on the site of the surgery, it may be necessary to obtain medical clearance before carrying out treatment.
SEVERE CIRCULATORY DISORDERS/ HEART CONDITION – always obtain medical clearance before treating a client with a severe heart condition or circulatory problem, as the increased circulation from the massage may overburden the heart and can increase the risk of thrombus or embolus.
- **THROMBOSIS/EMBOLISM** – there is a theoretical risk that a blood clot may become detached from its site of formation and be carried in the body to another part. Always refer to the client's GP for advice on the severity of the condition before offering treatment.
- **HIGH BLOOD PRESSURE** – clients with high blood pressure should have a medical referral prior to Indian Head Massage even in they are on prescribed medication, due to their susceptibility to form clots. Clients on anti-hypertensive drugs may be prone to postural hypotension and may feel light headed and dizzy after treatment. Therapists are advised to carefully monitor a client's reaction and advise clients to get up slowly after treatment. Massage is usually recommended to be soothing and relaxing.
LOW BLOOD PRESSURE – see above cautions under High Blood Pressure.
- **DYSFUNCTION OF THE NERVOUS SYSTEM** – clients with any dysfunction of the nervous system should be referred to their GP before treatment is given. A light relaxing massage may be indicated in the case of a client with Cerebral Palsy, Multiple Sclerosis or Parkinson's Disease, as massage may help to reduce spasms and involuntary movements and reduce rigidity and stiffness. Always seek medical advice before offering treatment.
- **EPILEPSY** – always refer to the client's GP regarding the type and nature of Epilepsy the client may suffer from. Caution is advised due to the complexity of this condition and the risk that deep relaxation or over stimulation could provoke a convulsion (although this has never been proven in practice). As some types of epilepsy may be triggered by smells, care should be taken with choice of oils or medium.
- **DIABETES** – this is a condition that requires medical referral, as clients with diabetes may be prone to arteriosclerosis, high blood pressure and oedema. Pressure should be carefully monitored due to any loss in sensory function resulting in the client being unable to give accurate feedback regarding pressure.

If the client is receiving insulin by injection, care should be taken to avoid massage on recent injection sites. Clients should have their necessary medications with them when they attend for treatment, in the event of an emergency.

CANCER – medical clearance should always be sought before massaging a client with cancer. It is unlikely that gentle massage can cause cancer to spread through the stimulation of lymph flow, however it is important to obtain advice from the Consultant/ medical team concerning the types of cancer and the extent of the disease.

If massage is indicated avoid massage over areas of the body receiving radiation therapy, close to tumour sites and areas of skin cancer.

Light massage can be beneficial in relaxing the client and supporting the immune system.

SKIN DISORDERS – care should be taken as the condition may be worsened. Some skin conditions such as eczema, dermatitis and psoriasis should be treated as a localised contra-indication as affected areas may be hypersensitive and the condition may be exacerbated by massage.

RECENT SCAR TISSUE – massage should only applied once the tissue is fully healed and can withstand pressure. Gentle frictions may be applied over healed scar tissue in order to help break down adhesions.

SEVERE BRUISING, OPEN CUTS OR ABRASIONS – these should be treated as localised contra-indications, and if present in the treatment areas they should be avoided.

UNDIAGNOSED LUMPS, BUMPS AND SWELLINGS – the client should be referred to their GP for a diagnosis. Massage may increase the susceptibility to damage in the area by virtue of pressure and motion.

Special factors to take into consideration before massaging and which may require additional care:

- **ALLERGIES** – care should be taken to ensure that any oils or products used do not contain items to which the client may be allergic. Patch tests should be carried out to avoid adverse reactions.
- **MEDICATION** – certain medications may inhibit or distort the client's response to give feedback regarding pressure, discomfort and pain. Always check with the client's GP if you are unsure as to type of medication and its effects.
- **MIGRAINE** – it is inadvisable to carry out treatment if a client indicates the onset of an attack of migraine due to the fact they may become nauseous, dizzy, experience visual disturbances with severe headache and possible vomiting. In reality, clients experiencing an acute attack of migraine will usually be incapacitated from its effects and would be unable to receive treatment, let alone desire a treatment, at the time of the attack. *However, Indian Head Massage may help as a preventative treatment, particularly if the migraine is stress induced.*

■ **PREGNANCY** – although pregnancy is not strictly a contra-indication, unless there are serious complications, special care should be taken with a pregnant client to ensure that they are comfortable during the treatment. Therapists should be aware that some women may experience side effects as a result of the pregnancy such as dizziness and high blood pressure. Pressure and duration of treatment may need to be adjusted according to the individual circumstances.

Below is an example of a Consultation form that may be used for Indian Head Massage

---

Indian Head Massage Consultation Form

Client Note

The following information is required for your safety and to benefit your health. Whilst Indian Head Massage is a very safe treatment, there are certain conditions which may require special attention.

The following information will be treated in the strictest of confidence and it may be necessary for you to consult your GP before treatment can be given.

Date of initial consultation: _____Client Ref. No. _____

Personal Details

Name: _____   Title: Mr/Mrs/Miss/Ms/Other _____

Address: _____

_____

Telephone Number: _____ (evening)   _____ (daytime)

Date of Birth: _____   Occupation: _____

Medical Details

Do you have / have you ever suffered with:

(please give dates and details)

			Dates and Details
High temperature or fever?	Y	N	_____
Acute infectious disease?	Y	N	_____
Skin infections?	Y	N	_____
Recent haemorrhage?	Y	N	_____
Are you currently under the influence of alcohol or drugs?	Y	N	_____
Recent head or neck injury?	Y	N	_____
Recent surgery?	Y	N	_____
Severe circulatory disorder?	Y	N	_____
Heart condition	Y	N	_____
Thrombosis / Embolism?	Y	N	_____
High or low blood pressure?	Y	N	_____
Dysfunction of the nervous system?	Y	N	_____
Epilepsy?	Y	N	_____
Diabetes?	Y	N	_____
Any potentially fatal / terminal condition?	Y	N	_____
Recent scar tissue?	Y	N	_____
Severe bruising, open cuts or abrasions?	Y	N	_____
Undiagnosed lumps, bumps or swellings?	Y	N	_____
Allergies?	Y	N	_____
Migraine or headaches?	Y	N	_____
Scalp infection?	Y	N	_____

Female Clients

Is it possible that you may be pregnant?	Y	N	_____
Are there any other conditions you have, which may affect the proposed treatment?	Y	N	_____

Details: _____

_____

_____

Are you currently taking any medication?   **Y ( )   N ( )**

Details (including dosages): _____

_____

Is GP referral required: Y ( )   N ( )

Clearance form sent: Y ( )   N ( ) Date _____

Clearance form received: Y ( )   N ( ) Date _____

Name of Doctor: _____   Surgery: _____

Address: _____

_____

Telephone Number: _____

Lifestyle

Is your general health / immunity: Good ( )   Average ( )   Poor ( )
Are your stress levels: High ( )   Medium ( )   Low ( )
Are your energy levels: High ( )   Medium ( )   Low ( )
Do you find time for relaxation / hobbies: Y ( )   N ( )

Details: _____

_____

Client Declaration

I declare that the information I have given is correct and as far as I am aware, I can undertake treatments without any adverse effects.

I have been fully informed about contra-indications and am therefore willing to proceed with treatment.

I understand that Indian Head Massage does not substitute medical treatment.

Client signature: _____Date: _____

LIASING WITH OTHER HEALTH CARE PROFESSIONALS

As the benefits of Indian Head Massage become more widely known and validated, there are more opportunities opening up for therapists to work alongside other health care professionals. Therapists therefore need to be aware of professional and medical etiquette when liasing with other professionals.

Referral to a Health Care Professional

If a contra-indication is established with a client at the time of consultation, treatment cannot usually proceed without reference to the client's GP. In this case, it is professional etiquette to have a pre-prepared referral form on headed notepaper that may be taken by the client to their Doctor or may be posted with a stamped addressed envelope. When referring to a client's GP it is essential that holistic therapists make it clear that they are seeking information about the client's medical condition in order to decide whether Indian Head Massage treatment is suitable and that their proposed treatment is in accordance with medical advice. In order to raise awareness of Indian Head Massage amongst health care professionals, it is important for a therapists to include literature on Indian Head Massage concerning its methodology, benefits and effects.

Handling Referral Data from other Health Care Professionals

If a client has been referred to them by another health care professional, it is professional etiquette to reply with a status report on the client's progress. Report writing is an essential part of networking with other professionals, as it helps to raise awareness of the benefits of the treatment and its value in a client's physical and emotional well-being. A status report should include the following information:

- A general introduction to the client and how he or she was referred
- A summary of the client's main presenting problems
- An evaluation of the therapist's findings
- The treatment used and explanation of the techniques involved
- The client's progress
- Recommendations for future/ continued treatment

The most important factor in the consultation besides whether the client is medically suitable for treatment, is their expectations and objectives of the treatment.

FORMULATING A TREATMENT PLAN FOR INDIAN HEAD MASSAGE

Once the verbal and non-verbal information has been elicited from the client, the therapist is then in a position to suggest a treatment plan or strategy and obtain the client's agreement before proceeding.

A treatment plan for Indian Head Massage will include the following information:
- The date of the treatment
- The treatment objectives and client expectations
- Any special considerations (such as specific areas to be worked on)
- The treatment duration
- Suggested treatment frequency (this may also be reviewed at the end of the treatment)
- Any mediums to be used (optional use of oils on the scalp)
- The client's agreement

> **KEY NOTE** An important consideration in a client's treatment plan may be the time of day the treatment is undertaken. A client may require the treatment in the morning to gently awaken the nerves and prepare the body for a day's activities or may require the appointment later to help remove the stresses of the day and promote sleep.

Important information to be recorded after the treatment includes:
- manual assessment of the client (noting any areas of tension, physiological responses)
- visual assessment of the client (noting posture, non-verbal signs)
- any known reactions
- after care advice
- home care advice – use of oils
- the results/ outcome of the treatment
- recommendations for future treatment

INDICATIONS FOR TREATMENT

There are many conditions which a client may present that may benefit from Indian Head Massage.

Common conditions Indian Head Massage has been known to help with include:
- Tension Headaches
- Eyestrain
- Muscular Tension
- Emotional Stress

■ Anxiety and Depression
■ Insomnia and disturbed sleep patterns
■ Sinusitis
■ Poor hair condition

CASE STUDY 1

Male Client
Civil Servant
49 years old
Very tall and large framed

INITIAL CONSULTATION

The client revealed that he had been receiving osteopathic treatment for a previous neck injury. However, the current condition of the client did not prove to be contra-indicated to treatment, although caution when treating the neck area was prudent. The client did not present with any other conditions or considerations for treatment, but had recently been experiencing high levels of stress due to recent personal circumstances.

TREATMENT OBJECTIVES

After consultation, it was agreed with the client that the treatment objectives were to:
■ Help relieve muscular tension in the shoulders and neck
■ Help relieve muscular tension generally, to aid relaxation
■ Help to uplift the client psychologically and aid stress relief

Account of Treatment

Over a 2 week period, the client received 3 treatments at regular intervals. During the treatments, care and lighter pressures were used in conjunction with the neck area. As the client was balding and had little hair, the treatments were adapted by applying light massage to the scalp, for the appropriate parts of the treatment routine.

The first treatment uncovered a lot of tension and proved to be slightly discomforting for the client in the region of the neck. The sinus area on the face also exhibited signs of puffiness, however the client enjoyed the treatment and felt relaxed at its conclusion.

During the second treatment, the client was visibly more relaxed and less tension was noticeable, the sinuses were less puffy and a greater relaxation was achieved at its conclusion.

During the third treatment, the client was commenting on the overall improvement he was experiencing. The muscular tension and pain was much improved and he was feeling extremely relaxed, yet much more positive and uplifted in his overall demeanour.

Outcomes and Recommendations

The series of treatments that this client has received have certainly proved to be beneficial. During and after each treatment, the improvements have been visibly noticeable. The client has himself commented enthusiastically on how much better he has felt and that the initial objectives have been achieved, even surpassed.

Further treatments are recommended in order to maintain the client's improvement and condition and in line with the client's request to continue the treatments. Recommended frequency would be once or twice a week, circumstances permitting, and then once or twice a fortnight in line with stress levels and tension build up.

CASE STUDY 2

Male Client
Technical Service Adviser
19 years old
Large framed

INITIAL CONSULTATION

The client was born with a hole in the heart and has medical checks every 2 years on his condition. He has not, and currently does not suffer with any other conditions medically which would prevent treatment, other than a recent viral infection. The infection has now dissipated but has left him feeling very tired and exhausted, particularly after activities such as when returning from work. He is normally very happy go lucky , but has felt low recently due to the tiredness he has been experiencing.

TREATMENT OBJECTIVES

After consultation, it was agreed with the client that the treatment objectives were to:

- Help strengthen his immune system and clear congestion
- Help aid relaxation and re-balance his body
- Help to psychologically uplift him

Account of Treatment

The client received 4 treatments at fairly regular intervals over a 2 month period.

During the first treatment, the client was twitchy with his head occasionally jerking. He commented on feeling in a hypnotised state, feeling very relaxed and tired and that his legs felt very heavy. After the treatment, he laid down for about ten minutes with a feeling of tiredness which was then replaced by a refreshed feeling.

Each treatment following the first, the client expressed an extreme tiredness of about 10 minutes after each treatment. This would then be replaced by a feeling of being wide eyed and fighting fit in the words of the client. Each treatment produced extreme relaxation within the client, followed by a profound change in state about 10 minutes after each treatment. The client felt better at work with even his colleagues commenting on how much more alert and talkative he appeared.

Outcomes and Recommendations

The treatments have proved to have been very successful for this client; he has stated that since commencing the treatments, he has felt so much better, the congested feeling in his head and the sluggish feelings that he experienced now seem to have disappeared. He has requested to continue to have treatments for body maintenance and relaxation. Suggested frequency for treatments would be weekly or as client desires in line with state of health.

CASE STUDY 3

Female Client
Accountant
27 years old
Average height / small framed

INITIAL CONSULTATION

This client has a history of very painful periods which has caused her to undergo surgery in the past. She still suffers from bad migraines and stomach pains for which she takes medication. She also gets very drained and suffers low energy levels due to having to cope with her menstrual-related symptoms each month.

TREATMENT OBJECTIVES

After consultation, it was agreed with the client that the treatment objectives were to:
- promote psychological uplift
- aid relaxation
- help relieve tension
- help against headaches

Account of Treatment

Over a period of 17 days, the client received 3 treatments at regular intervals.

During the first treatment, a lot of tension was found in the head and neck areas, the neck was very tight and the head very stiff. A lot of deep breathing was suggested to help ease the tension during the treatment. The client later confirmed that she did suffer with a lot of neck ache, but commented on her surprise at how relaxed the treatment had made her feel.

At the second treatment, the client stated that she had suffered headaches and tiredness since her first treatment. She was also currently experiencing menstrual pains and found this treatment to be uncomfortable and tended to fidget throughout the treatment.

By the third treatment, the client again reported feelings of tiredness since her last treatment and was feeling low and a little stressed from work. She did however comment on how enjoyable she finds some of the techniques and that they do help to relax her.

Outcomes and Recommendations

Although not much improvement was noted in the condition of the client or indicated by the client, it would appear that the treatments had at least been beneficial to a certain degree. Tension which was initially detected in the client did decrease at each treatment. The client also indicated her gradual enjoyment and relaxation.

Further treatments would be recommended initially as frequent as twice or three times a week. The client's improvement would possibly be slow, hence the frequent treatments. However, Indian Head Massage would certainly help as part of an overall programme to combat the problems she is experiencing.

Client Consultation
Self Assessment Questions

1. What important skills does a therapist need to carry out an effective consultation for Indian Head Massage treatment?

2. State 3 conditions for which Indian Head Massage is contra-indicated, stating why in each case

3. State 3 conditions which should be referred to a GP before treatment is offered. State why in each case

4. State 5 important factors that should be discussed with a client during a consultation for Indian Head Massage

5. List the important information which should be recorded on a client's treatment plan for Indian Head Massage treatment

CHAPTER 4

Conditions Affecting the Head, Neck and Shoulders

A considerable increase in stress levels in the sophisticated present day life, has led to a great deal of interest in holistic therapies such as Indian Head Massage, which continues to grow in popularity. More and more people are seeking the benefits of an Indian Head Massage treatment to help improve their emotional and physical well-being.

Therapists practising Indian Head Massage need to be knowledgeable within the sphere of their chosen therapy, but also be sufficiently familiar with conditions affecting the head, neck and shoulders in order to design a safe and effective treatment plan that is adapted to the client's needs.

By the end of this chapter, you will be able to relate the following to your practical work:

- ■ Knowledge of common conditions of the head, neck and shoulders
- ■ The cautions, recommendations and restrictions involved in treatment application

This knowledge will help to empower therapists to make an informed decision as to a suitable treatment plan that is within safe and ethical medical guidelines. It is very important that a therapist never diagnoses a client's medical condition, and refers the client to their GP before any form of treatment is commenced.

> **KEY NOTE** It should be noted that whilst the information given reflects an accurate representation of the condition in generic terms, all clients will vary in the severity of their condition. Each client should be individually assessed as to their condition at the time of the proposed treatment and re-assessed on subsequent treatments. The guidelines given are meant as a general guide and thus therapists are encouraged to seek further clarification of a client's medical condition from the GP and from the client themselves.

Alopecia

A term used to describe temporary baldness, or severe hair loss which may follow illness, shock, a period of extreme stress, or may be the side effect of drug therapy (i.e. chemotherapy). It is important to distinguish temporary baldness from male pattern baldness which is progressive and permanent and is unlikely to be helped by therapies such as Indian Head Massage.

Patchy hair loss, or Alopecia areata is a relatively common disorder. The onset is fairly sudden and presents with an round or oval bald area; the loss of hair may be complete or so-called 'exclamation mark hairs' may be seen in the bald patches or at the edges. Occasionally the scalp is erythematous (red) in the part affected. The skin itself is not scaly as opposed to bald areas seen in fungus infection of the scalp.

In Alopecia areata there may be one or several bald patches. The most frequent course for alopecia areata to take is for the hair to regrow after a period of time (frequently two to three months). When regrowth occurs the hair is often white but usually repigments in time.

Cautions, restrictions and recommendations

- Concentrate on massaging the scalp to increase the local circulation using almond or coconut oil
- Wrap a warm towel round the head after the treatment to help aid the absorption
- Encourage client to use the oils and massage the scalp at home twice a week leaving the oils to absorb for about two hours before shampooing
- Advise client of the importance of dietary requirements for healthy hair (adequate protein and essential fatty acids to promote healthy growth, and vitamin B complex and vitamin C to provide nourishment for the hair follicles, Vitamin B5 helps to relieve stress)

Angina

Pain in the left side of the chest and usually radiating to the left arm. Caused by insufficient blood to the heart muscle; usually on exertion or excitement. The pain is often described as constricting or suffocating, which can last for a few seconds or moments. Patient may become pale and sweaty. This condition indicates ischaemic heart disease.

Cautions, restrictions and recommendations

- As stress predisposes an angina attack, Indian Head Massage can help to reduce stress levels by reducing the activity of the sympathetic nervous system
- As sudden exposure to extreme heat or cold can bring on an attack, keep the client warm and avoid extreme fluctuations in temperature
- It is important that clients have their necessary medications with them when they attend for treatment, in the event of an emergency

Ankylosing spondylitis

A systemic joint disease characterised by inflammation of the intervertebral disc spaces, costo-vertebral and sacroiliac joints. Fibrosis, calcification, ossification and stiffening of joints are common and the spine becomes rigid. Typically, a client will complain of persistent or intermittent lower back pain. Kyphosis is present when the thoracic or cervical regions of the spine are affected and the weight of the head compresses the vertebrae and bends the spine forward. This condition can cause muscular atrophy, loss of balance and falls. Typically Ankylosing spondylitis affects young male adults.

Cautions, restrictions and recommendations

- Position the client according to individual comfort – extra cushioning and support may be required
- Avoid forcibly mobilising ankylosed joints, and in the case of cervical spondylitis avoid hyperextending the neck
- Gentle massage may be very beneficial as the heat generated may help to ease the pain.
- Advise the client to do breathing exercises regularly in order to help mobilise the thorax

Anxiety

This can be defined as fear of the unknown, but as an illness it can vary from a mild form to panic attacks and severe phobias that can be disabling socially, psychologically and at times physically.

It presents with feeling of dread that something serious is likely to happen and is associated with palpitations, rapid breathing, sweaty hands, tremor (shakiness), dry mouth, general indigestion, feeling of butterflies in the stomach, occasional diarrhoea and generalised aches and pains in the muscles. It can present with similar features of mild to moderate depression of the agitated type. The causes of anxiety can be related to personality with some genetic and behavioural predisposition, or a traumatic experience or physical illness i.e. hyperthyroidism.

- Clients are likely to present with various symptoms and therefore a thorough assessment is required
- Indian Head Massage and relaxation exercises are likely to be a valuable source of help and support
- Clients with anxiety are more likely to become emotionally dependent on their therapist and may need to be referred to another professional for help

Arthritis – Osteoarthritis

A joint disease characterised by the breakdown of articular cartilage, growth of bony spikes, swelling of the surrounding synovial membrane and stiffness and tenderness of the joint. Is also known as degenerative arthritis.

It is common in the elderly and takes a progressive course.

This condition involves varying degrees of joint pain, stiffness, limitation of movement, joint instability and deformity.

It commonly affects the weight bearing joints – the hips, knees, the lumbar and cervical vertebrae.

Cautions, restrictions and recommendations

- Passive and gentle friction movements around the joint may be beneficial where there is minimal pain, but excessive movement may cause joint pain and damage
- Gentle massage may help with muscle spasms, joint stiffness and muscle atrophy
- Always ask the client to demonstrate the range of movement possible in their shoulder and their neck; this will guide you as to the limitations of treatment possible

Arthritis – Rheumatoid

Chronic inflammation of peripheral joints resulting in pain, stiffness and potential damage to joints. It can cause severe disability. Joint swellings and rheumatoid nodules are tender.

Cautions, restrictions and recommendations

- Although Indian Head Massage cannot cure arthritis, it can help to prevent its progress through relaxation and reduction of discomfort
- In the early stages of diagnosis, clients should be encouraged to have treatment in order to maintain the range of joint movements and help prevent contractures
- In the acute stage, avoid massaging but encourage passive movement of the affected joints. In the chronic stage treatments, massage movements can help to reduce the thickening that occurs in and around the articular cartilage
- Always ensure there is no pain and that care is taken when gently mobilising a joint
- Treatment is generally of shorter duration as clients may be taking painkillers and be unable to give adequate feedback

Asthma

A condition in which there are attacks of shortness of breath and difficulty in breathing due to spasm or swelling of the bronchial tubes, caused by hypersensitivity to allergens such as pollens of various plants, grass, flowers, pet hair, dust mites and various proteins in foodstuffs such as shellfish, eggs and milk. Asthma may be exacerbated by exercise, anxiety, stress or smoking. It runs in families and can be associated with Hayfever and Eczema.

Cautions, restrictions and recommendations

- Indian Head Massage is ideally suited as a treatment for asthma sufferers as clients are seated in an upright position

- Always obtain a detailed history during the consultation stage, specifically the triggers that bring on an attack. If the client has a history of allergies then ensure the client is not allergic to any preparations or substances you may be proposing to use
- Relaxation provided by the treatment along with deep breathing exercises can help to reduce bronchiospasm and should be encouraged
- It is advisable for the client to have their required medications handy, in the event of an attack

Bells Palsy

A disorder of the 7th cranial nerve (facial nerve) that results in paralysis on one side of the face. The disorder usually comes on suddenly and is commonly caused by inflammation around the facial nerve as it travels from brain to the exterior.

It may be caused by pressure on the nerve due to tumours, injury to the nerve, infection of the meninges or inner ear, or dental surgery. Diabetes, pregnancy and hypertension are other causes.

The condition may present with a drooping of the mouth on the affected side due to flaccid paralysis of the facial muscles and there may be difficulty in puckering the lips due to paralysis of the orbicularis oris muscle. Taste may be diminished or lost if the nerve has been affected proximal to the branch, which carries taste sensations. The condition also presents with the individual having difficulty in closing the eye tightly and creasing the forehead. The buccinator muscle is also affected which prevents the client from puffing the cheeks and is the cause of food getting caught between the teeth and cheeks. There is also excessive tearing from the affected eye. Pain may be present near the angle of the jaw and behind the ear.

Eighty to ninety per cent of individuals recover spontaneously and completely in around 1-8 weeks. Corticosteriods may be used to reduce the inflammation of the nerve.

Cautions, restrictions and recommendations

- Be aware that cold and chills are known to trigger Bells Palsy
- Use light strokes in an upward direction from the middle of the face to the sides (towards the ears)
- To help increase tone on the affected side of the face, use kneading movements with the finger tips
- Light tapotement (tapping) and vibration movements may be used to help stimulate paralysed muscles
- To help maintain tone, the face massage can be performed two to three times a day
- The client may also be shown facial exercises:
  (i) To exercise the orbicularis oculi ask the client to alternately close and open the eyes with and without mild resistance to the eyelids
  (ii) To exercise the buccinator ask the client to puff the cheeks put and in and then try and whistle

(iii) To exercise the orbicularis oris the mouth should be puckered

(iv) Saying the words P,B,M,N helps to exercise the labials

(v) To exercise the frontalis muscle ask the client to raise and lower the eyebrows

- Electrotherapy (non-surgical face lift machines or faradic) may be used to reduce the atrophy of the affected muscles

Bronchitis

A chronic or acute inflammation of the bronchial tubes. Chronic Bronchitis is common in smokers and may lead to emphysema, which is caused by damage to lung structure. Acute Bronchitis can result from a recent cold or flu.

Cautions, restrictions and recommendations

- Clients with Bronchitis may find Indian Head Massage more comfortable due to the fact they are seated
- Encourage the client to breathe slowly and deeply throughout the treatment
- As sufferers of chronic bronchitis are prone to respiratory infection, therapists should avoid treating such clients if they have even the mildest form of acute chest infection

Cerebral Palsy

A condition caused by damage to the central nervous system, of the baby during pregnancy, delivery or soon after birth. The damage could be due to bleeding, lack of oxygen or other injuries to the brain. The signs and symptoms of this condition depend on the area of the brain affected.

Speech is impaired in most individuals and there may be difficulty in swallowing. There may or may not be mental retardation.

Muscles may increase in tone to become spastic, making co-ordinated movements difficult. The muscles are hyperexcitable and even small movements, touch, stretch of muscle or emotional stress can increase the spasticity.

The posture is abnormal due to muscle spacticity and the gait is also affected. Some may have abnormal involuntary movements of the limbs that may be exaggerated on voluntarily performing a task. Weakness of muscles may also be associated with the condition, along with seizures. There may also be problems with hearing and vision.

Cautions, restrictions and recommendations

- Seek the support of the doctors, nurses, physiotherapist and the family before proceeding
- Indian Head Massage can help to reduce stress, prevent contractures, improve the circulation to the skin and muscles that are unused and provide tremendous emotional support

- Perform a shorter treatment (15-20 minutes) using mild to moderate pressure
- Since any form of stress increases the symptoms, concentrate on relaxation as this will help to reduce muscular spasms and involuntary movements
- Be aware that some clients may have reduced sensations and due to mental retardation may be unable to give adequate feedback regarding pressure and pain
- Also be aware that the spasticity in an individual may change from day to day, with changes in posture and is related to emotional stress

Dandruff (Pityriasis capitis)

An extremely common condition which presents with visible scaling from the surface of the scalp and is associated with the presence of the yeast Pityrosporum ovale. It is the precursor of seborrhoeic eczema of the scalp, in which there is a degree of inflammation in addition to the greasy scaling.

Cautions, restrictions and recommendations

- Place a clean towel over the client's shoulders when proceeding to the scalp massage, to prevent dead skin cells from the scalp falling onto their clothing
- Regular scalp massage and use of oils helps to remove dead skin cells and increase the circulation
- Vitamin A is useful for a dry, scaly scalp

Depression

This combines symptoms of lowered mood, loss of appetite, poor sleep, lack of concentration and interest, lack of sense of enjoyment, occasional constipation and loss of libido. There are occasions when there is suicidal thinking, death wish or active suicide attempts.

Depression can be the result of chemical imbalance, usually related to serotonin and noradrenalin. The cause of depression could be endogenous where there is no cause for depression, but is thought to be linked to genetic predisposition, the result of physical illness, actual loss of a close relative, object, limb or loss of a relationship.

A depressed person looks miserable, hunchbacked, downcast and will usually avoid eye contact.

The severity, as suggested above, can be variable but may become severe enough to become psychotic manifested by hallucinations, delusions, paranoia or thought disorders.

Cautions, restrictions and recommendations

- A depressed client can present with physical ailments including back ache, gastro-intestinal symptoms (usually constipation) and headaches
- Physical illness can present with depression and can include long term illness, terminal illness, Parkinson's disease and arthritis for instance

- Therapists need to ensure that clients do not become emotionally dependent on them; they may need to be referred to another Professional
- If there is any inclination of suicidal thinking at any time, the client should be referred to their GP
- Indian Head Massage is thought to help increase levels of serotonin from the brain and may be effective in helping to lift depression

Epilepsy

A neurological disorder that makes the individual susceptible to recurrent and temporary seizures. Epilepsy is a complex condition and classifications of types of epilepsy are not definitive.

GENERALISED – this may take the form of major or tonic-clinic seizures (formerly known as grand mal) in which, at the onset the patient falls to the ground unconscious with their muscles in a state of spasm (tonic phase). This is then replaced by convulsive movements (the clonic phase) when the tongue may be bitten and urinary incontinence may occur. Movements gradually cease and the patient may rouse in a state of confusion, complaining of a headache or may fall asleep.

PARTIAL – this may be idiopathic or a symptom of structural damage to the brain. In one type of partial idiopathic epilepsy, often affecting children, seizures may take the form of absences (formerly known as petit mal), in which there are brief spells of unconsciousness lasting for a few seconds. The eyes stare blankly and there may be fluttering movements of the lids and momentary twitching of the fingers and mouth. This form of epilepsy seldom appears before the age of three or after adolescence. It often subsides spontaneously in adult life, but may be followed by the onset of generalised or partial epilepsy.

FOCAL – this is partial epilepsy due to brain damage (either local or due to a stroke). The nature of the seizure depends on the location of the damage in the brain. In a Jacksonian motor seizure the convulsive movements may spread from the thumb to the hand, arm and face.

PSYCHOMOTOR – this type of epilepsy is caused by dysfunction of the cortex of the temporal lobe of the brain. Symptoms may include hallucinations of smell, taste, sight and hearing. Throughout an attack the patient is in a state of clouded awareness and afterwards may have no recollection of the event.

Cautions, restrictions and recommendations

- Always refer to the client's GP regarding the type and nature of Epilepsy
- As Epilepsy is a complex condition and head massage involves stimulation of the brain, caution is advised
- If on controlled medication, the chances of a seizure are minimal, however caution is advised due to the complexity of this condition
- It has never been reported that holistic therapies have ever provoked the onset of epilepsy, although there is a theoretical risk to be considered in that deep relaxation or over stimulation could provoke an attack (although this has never been proven in practice)

Fibromyalgia

A chronic condition that produces musculo-skeletal pain. Predominant symptoms include widespread musculoskeletal pain, lethargy and fatigue. Other characteristic features include a non-refreshing sleep pattern in which the patient feels exhausted and more tired than later in the day and interrupted sleep. Other recognised symptoms include early morning stiffness, pins and needles sensation, unexplained headaches, poor concentration, memory loss, low mood, urinary frequency, abdominal pain, irritable bowel syndrome. Anxiety and depression are also common.

Cautions, restrictions and recommendations

- Avoid deep massage on localised tender areas (which include base of skull, cervical vertebrae C5-7, midpoint of the upper border of the trapezius, above the spine of the scapula)
- Caution is advised regarding stiffness
- Relaxation is integral to reduce muscle spasm and reduce feeling of stress

Frozen Shoulder (adhesive capsulitis)

A chronic condition in which there is pain and stiffness and reduced mobility, or locking, of the shoulder joint. This may follow an injury, a stroke or myocardial infarction or may develop due to incorrect lifting or a sudden movement.

Cautions, restrictions and recommendations

If the condition is severe, refer the client to a Physiotherapist. Avoid massaging the affected areas whilst there is acute inflammation. This condition can cause neck pain and pain at the base of the skull, which results in a headache.

Be aware that the synovial capsule of shoulder joint will be tender and surrounding muscles and tendons will also be affected. The client will benefit from gentle stretching exercises to help mobilise the shoulder joint.

Headache (Tension)

This is the most common type of headache. It involves contraction and spasm of the neck and scalp muscles. The pain is produced by the pressure of the contracted muscle on the nerves and blood vessels in the area. The resultant blood flow increases the accumulation of waste products (such as lactic acid) in the area which perpetuate the pain.

The sufferer will usually complain of a dull, persistent ache and a feeling of tightness around the head, temple, forehead and occiput. Factors that may precipitate an attack include mental strain, noise, bright lights, alcohol consumption, menstruation and fatigue.

Cautions, restrictions and recommendations

- It is important to try and identify the precipitating cause of the headache
- Indian Head Massage is usually very successful in helping to relieve this type of headache, particularly if it is stress induced
- Encourage the client to relax the shoulder and neck muscles with relaxation exercises before commencing the massage
- Concentrate on relaxing areas that are less tense with effleurage (smoothing/stroking) and gentle kneading and then move onto muscles which are in spasm with frictions (it is likely that these will be the neck muscles, trapezius, levator scapula and the rhomboids)
- Massage of the scalp and face can be helpful (concentrating on the temporalis muscle, the masseters and the frontalis)
- Remember that clients may be taking pain killers and therefore may give inadequate feedback

Kyphosis

A deformity of the spine that produces a rounded back. The condition presents with a rounded back and a flattened chest. There may be difficulty in breathing due to shortening of the pectoral muscles and the back muscle become weakened. In this condition the scapula tends to be pulled forward and the head is pushed forward.

Cautions, restrictions and recommendations

- A postural assessment is required in order to identify range of motion
- Take care with the positioning of the client and if necessary offer supporting cushions/pillows
- Concentrate on relaxing the muscles of the shoulders and neck
- Gentle stretching exercises for the back and neck may help to improve posture
- The aim of the treatment will be to relax and reduce pain in tense muscles
- Deep diaphragmatic breathing should be encouraged to help mobilise the thorax
- Avoid joint mobilisation if the condition is due to changes in bone or connective tissue

Migraine

Specific form of headache, usually unilateral (one side of the head), associated with nausea or vomiting, visual disturbances usually scintillating light waves or zigzag fashion. Client may experience a visual aura before an attack actually happens. This is usually called a Classical Migraine. On occasions they cause painful, red and watery eyes – Ophthalmoplegic Migraine.

Another form of migraine can cause one sided paralysis. Weakness of the face and body, called Neuropathic Migraine.

Abdominal Migraine can affect children which present with recurring attacks of abdominal pain with or without nausea/ vomiting.

Migraine can be treated with simple analgesia to more specialised anti-migraine medication.

Cautions, restrictions and recommendations

- Avoid treatment during acute attacks and especially if the condition has not yet been diagnosed
- Indian Head Massage is well known in helping migraine sufferers, as the relaxation and relief from stress and tension can help reduce frequency of attacks
- Remember that women are likely to have more attacks during premenstrual periods, when they are taking contraceptive pill, during the menopause or when starting HRT
- Tension headaches can be a variant of migraine. Indian Head Massage is an ideal therapy in this event

Myalgic encephalomyelitis (Chronic fatigue syndrome)

A condition which is characterised by extreme disabling fatigue that has lasted for at least six months and is made worse by physical or mental exertion and is not resolved by bed rest. The symptom of fatigue is often accompanied by some of the following; muscle pain or weakness, poor co-ordination, joint pain, slight fever, sore throat, painful lymph nodes in the neck and armpits, depression, inability to concentrate and general malaise.

It can happen in any age group, but recently children and adolescents are noticed to have a higher incidence.

Cautions, restrictions and recommendations

- This is a condition which can benefit from Indian Head Massage, but avoid any claim which could be misinterpreted as curative
- Relaxation can help the client to cope
- Be aware of tenderness in the muscle and joints
- Clients may require a lot of support and understanding

Multiple Sclerosis

Disease of the central nervous system, in which the myelin (fatty) sheath covering the nerve fibres is destroyed and various functions become impaired, including movement and sensations. Multiple sclerosis is characterised by relapses and remissions. It can present with blindness or reduced vision and can lead to severe disability within a short period. It can also cause incontinence, loss of balance, tremor and speech problems. Depression and mania can happen.

Cautions, restrictions and recommendations

- Be aware of loss of sensation
- Be aware that massage and joint movement may trigger muscle spasm

- Relaxation therapies and exercises may be helpful in decreasing tone in rigid muscles and preventing stiffness and contractures
- Temperature extremes may make the symptoms worse
- Treatments should be slow and gentle and of short duration as clients may tire easily

Psoriasis (of the Scalp)

A chronic skin disease which presents as erythematous (red) scaly lesions on the scalp (other common areas affected include the knees, elbows, hands, nails and the sacral area). The client with psoriasis of the scalp may complain of a severe case of dandruff. However, unlike dandruff scalp psoriasis can be easily felt as thick plaques occurring in patches. It may cause some hair thinning which tends to recover with successful treatment of the psoriasis.

Cautions, restrictions and recommendations

See Pityriasis capitis

Caution is advised regarding the application of oils – avoid oils which are too hot or too stimulating to the scalp (almond and coconut are good choices). Acute flare-up of psoriasis can caused painful and tender lesions of skin and care is needed during massage. As psychological stress is a considerable cause in the exacerbation of psoriasis, Indian Head Massage can help clients to cope with their condition.

Seborrheic Eczema (or Dermatitis)

This condition presents with redness and diffuse scaling of the scalp (dandruff – see pityriasis capitis) which may be mild or severe. Red scaly areas may also occur on the face, especially in the eyebrows and the naso-labial folds. A similar rash may occur behind the ears.

Cautions, restrictions and recommendations

See Pityriasis capitis and Psoriasis of the Scalp

Sinusitis

A condition involving inflammation of the paranasal sinuses. It is usually caused by a viral or bacterial infection or may be associated with a common cold or allergy. The congestion of the nose results in a blockage in the opening of the sinus into the nasal cavity and a build up of pressure in the sinus.

The condition presents with nasal congestion followed by a mucous discharge from the nose. The pain is located to specific areas depending on the sinuses affected. If the frontal sinuses are affected, a major symptom is a headache over one or both eyes. If the maxillary sinuses are affected, one or both cheeks will hurt and is may feel as if there is a toothache in the upper jaw.

Cautions, restrictions and recommendations

■ Be aware of the sites of inflammation where there will be pain and swelling
■ Pressures around the eyes and around the zygomatic bones can help to drain the sinuses and help relieve pain
■ Encourage the client to drink plenty of water after the treatment to increase elimination and to consider a cleansing diet

Stroke

A blocking of blood flow to the brain by an embolus in a cerebral blood vessel. A stroke can result in a sudden attack of weakness affecting one side of the body, due to the interruption to the flow of blood to the brain. A stroke can vary in severity from a passing weakness or tingling in a limb to a profound paralysis and a coma if severe. Sometimes the term is used to describe cerebral haemorrhage when an artery or congenital cyst of blood vessels in the brain burst, resulting in damage to the brain and causing similar signs to thrombus of cerebral vessels. Haemorrhage is usually associated with severe headaches and can cause neck stiffness.

Cautions, restrictions and recommendations

■ Therapists will normally deal with clients who have recovered or are recovering from a stroke and Indian Head Massage can benefit and aid recovery
■ Be aware of muscle spasm and jerking movements in a paralysed limb
■ Neck massage is best avoided

Temporo-mandibular joint tension (TMJ syndrome)

A collection of symptoms and signs produced by disorders of the temporomandibular joint. It is characterised by bilateral or unilateral muscle tenderness and reduced motion. It presents with a dull aching pain around the joint often radiating to the ear, face, neck or shoulder. The condition may start off as clicking sounds in the joint. There may be protrusion of the jaw or hypermobility and pain on opening the jaw. It slowly progresses to decreased mobility of the jaw and locking of the jaw may occur.

Causes include chewing gum, biting nails, biting off large chunks of food, habitual protrusion of the jaw, tension in the muscles of the neck and back and clenching of the jaw. It may also be caused by injury and trauma to the joint or through a whiplash injury.

Cautions, restrictions and recommendations

■ Be aware that the masseter, temporalis and pterygoid muscles may be in spasms and will be tender
■ The muscles of the neck, base of skull and shoulders should be massaged thoroughly to help reduce tension and spasms

- The client needs to be educated on relaxing the muscles of the jaw. Ask the client to clench the jaw firmly and concentrate the feeling of tightness in the jaw, then relax and let the jaw fall open
- Clients may benefit from a posture assessment and breathing exercises
- Clients should be encouraged to consult their Dentist and a Physiotherapist for specific treatment techniques

Tinnitis

A condition where there is the sensation of sounds in the ears or head in the absence of an external sound source. The most common cause is ordinary age-related hair cell loss in the cochlear. Other causes include wax blocking the ear canal, damage to the ear drum, diseases of the inner ear such as Menieres Disease, and abnormalities of the auditory nerve.

Cautions, restrictions and recommendations

- Indian Head Massage has been known to be effective in clearing congestion in the head and may help relieve the symptoms
- Concentrate on relaxing the neck muscle and work thoroughly above, in front of and behind the ears to increase lymph drainage
- Be aware that some clients may experience dizziness and loss of balance upon rising

Trigemenal Neuralgia

A painful condition caused by irritation of the 5th cranial nerve (the trigemenal nerve).

The condition is characterised by excruciating intermittent pain confined to one or both sides of the face, along the distribution of the trigemenal nerve. The pain may be triggered by any touch or movement such as eating, chewing, swallowing etc. Exposure to hot or cold may also trigger an attack. Some cases of Facial Neuralgia are caused by shingles which has healed, leaving a potentially life-long pain.

Cautions, restrictions and recommendations

- Obtain a detailed history of the signs and symptoms and refer the client to their GP before proceeding
- The client may not allow you to touch the affected side of the face
- If the client finds massage beneficial, use smoothing movements and light frictions over the skull. Then stroke gently from the middle of the face towards the temples, starting in the least sensitive area and moving gradually towards the more sensitive areas
- Do not overwork the area as it may irritate the nerve and induce pain and discomfort
- Treatment may be scheduled every other day initially

Whiplash

A condition produced by damage to the muscles, ligaments, intervertebral discs or nerve tissues of the cervical region by sudden hyperextension and/or flexion of the neck.

The most common cause is a road traffic accident when acceleration/ deceleration causes sudden stretch of the tissue around the cervical spine. It may also occur as a result of hard impact sports. It can present with pain, limitation of neck movements with muscle tenderness which can start hours to days after the accident, and may take months to recover. This is usually affected by complicated physical, psychological and legal issues.

Cautions, restrictions and recommendations

- The condition may last for a few months or many years
- Consider compensation as a reason for delayed healing and therefore avoid making any comments about reasons, prognosis or suitability of the therapy
- Ascertain that the client is not seeking a cure; neither should the client receive any promise of doing so
- Take care when massaging the neck and avoid manipulation or moving vigorously
- Relaxation exercises can help
- Holistic therapies such as Indian Head Massage may help clients to cope with the condition
- Remember that clients with this condition would have seen many professionals and there may be legal issues you may want to avoid becoming involved with

Conditions affecting the Head, Neck and Shoulders

Self Assessment Questions

1. Describe how you would adapt a treatment plan for a client with the following conditions:

a) Alopecia

b) Dandruff (Pityriasis capitis)

c) Frozen Shoulder (Adhesive Capsulitis)

d) Osteoarthritis of the Neck

e) Psoriasis of the Scalp

CHAPTER 5

Maintaining and Supporting Employment Standards

Competency in the workplace requires a therapist to support standards in the workplace, in order to maintain employment. The success of a therapist lies not only in their ability to perform their own job roles effectively but to be able to contribute to the overall efficiency and operation of a business, upon which their livelihood ultimately depends. This chapter provides an overview of the employment standards required to support workplace practices.

By the end of this chapter you will be able to understand and apply the following knowledge to your workplace practice:

- The importance of appearance to enhance image of the workplace
- Hygiene precautions required for professional practice of Indian Head Massage
- The implications of relevant legislation in relation to Indian Head Massage
- The importance of good communication skills and maintaining workplace records to maintain efficient operation and services

THERAPIST'S APPEARANCE

A therapist practising Indian Head Massage should maintain a smart and hygienic working appearance at all times in order to project the right professional image of themselves and the establishment in which they are working. Attention should be paid to the following:

CLOTHING – specific workwear should be worn when practising Indian Head Massage to maintain hygiene and to project a professional image. Workwear should be clean, freshly laundered and ironed.

FOOTWEAR – when practising Indian Head Massage footwear should be low-heeled, comfortable, clean and of smart and professional appearance, i.e. trainers do not portray a professional appearance.

HAIR – should be clean, neatly styled and away from the face. It is important to tie long hair back for hygienic and practical reasons.

JEWELLERY AND ACCESSORIES – ideally no jewellery or accessories should be worn when massaging; specific attention is drawn to watches or rings and bracelets that may scratch or irritate a client's skin.

HANDS – these should be kept as soft as possible and protected from harsh chemicals. Nails must be kept short and without nail enamel.

PERSONAL HYGIENE – due to the close nature of an Indian Head Massage treatment, attention should be closely paid to maintaining personal hygiene to avoid offending a client with bad breath and body odour.

Health, Safety and Hygiene in the Workplace

Part of the role of a therapist is in following health, safety and hygiene regulations in order to develop safe working practices for themselves, their colleagues and their clients. In order to ensure a healthy, safe and secure working environment, a therapist must ensure that their work activities meet hygiene and safety requirements.

MAINTAINING A HYGIENIC AND SAFE WORKING ENVIRONMENT

Health and Safety is a broad term that also covers hygiene precautions. When practising Indian Head Massage attention should be paid to the following:

Safe working Conditions

- Premises, furnishings and fittings should be maintained in a safe condition and kept hygienically clean and neat at all times
- The work areas should be well-lit, particularly in stairways and fire escapes

- There should be adequate heating – a comfortable working temperature of 20-23 degrees Centigrade (68-75 degrees Fahrenheit)
- There should be adequate ventilation to keep the air smelling fresh and prevent buildup of fumes
- There should be a constant supply of hot and cold water and adequate sanitary facilities
- Any potential dangers in the workplace should be reported to the Supervisor of Manager for remedial action

Hygiene Precautions

- All equipment should be disinfected regularly
- Rubbish should be disposed of regularly in a sealed bin
- Open cuts or abrasions should be covered with a waterproof plaster
- All jewellery should be removed from the client and the therapist (with the exception of a wedding band)
- All materials and consumables used should be clean and hygienic, ensuring all tops are secured tightly after use
- Therapists hands should be washed with an anti-bacterial soap/hand cleanser before and after each client

> **KEY NOTE** Therapists practising Indian Head Massage in the workplace may benefit from using anti-bacterial dry hand cleansers if there are no facilities for washing hands nearby.

LEGISLATION

HEALTH, SAFETY AND HYGIENE is of paramount importance in the workplace. The law demands that every place of employment is a healthy, and above all safe place not only for employees to work in, but for their clients and other visitors who may enter the workplace.

Failure to comply with legislation may have serious consequences such as:
- claims from injured staff or clients
- loss of trade through bad publicity
- closure of the business

Health and Safety at Work Act 1974

The Health and Safety at Work Act provides a comprehensive legal framework to promote and encourage high standards of health and safety in the workplace.

The Health and Safety at Work Act covers a range of legislation relating to health and safety and both the employer and employee have responsibilities under the Act. If there are more than five employees a written Health and Safety Policy is required.

The Responsibilities of the Employer

- safeguard as far as possible the health, safety and welfare of themselves, their employees, contractors, employees and members of the public
- keep all equipment up to Health and Safety standards
- have safety equipment checked regularly
- ensure the environment is free from toxic fumes
- ensure that all staff are aware of safety procedures, by providing safety information and training
- ensure safe systems of work

The Responsibilities of the Employee

- adhere to the workplace rules and regulations concerning safety
- follow safe working practices and attending training as required
- take reasonable care to avoid injury to themselves and others
- co-operate with others in all matters relating to health and safety
- not interfere or wilfully misuse anything provided to protect their health and safety

> **KEY NOTE** The Health and Safety Executive (HSE) have produced a guide to the laws on Health & Safety and it is a requirement than an employer displays a copy of this poster in the workplace.

Electricity at Work Regulations 1989

Regulations under this Legislation are concerned with safety in connection the use of electricity. It is recommended that electrical equipment be checked regularly (at least once a year) by a competent person such as a qualified electrician or the local electricity board. All checks should be listed in a record book, stating the results of the tests and the recommendations and action taken in the case of defects. In the case of legal action, a record book may serve as important evidence. The checks that should be made in connection with electrical equipment include checking the fusing, insulation and that there are no loose or frayed wires.

The Personal Protective Equipment at Work Regulations 1992

This legislation requires an employer to:

- provide suitable protective clothing and equipment for all employees to ensure safety in the workplace
- ensure staff are adequately trained in the use of chemicals and equipment
- ensure that equipment is suitable for its purpose and is kept in a good state of repair

Control of Substances Hazardous to Health (COSHH) 1998

Regulations under this Legislation require employers to regulate employees' exposure to hazardous substances which may cause ill health or injury in the workplace and involves risk assessment. Risk assessment involves making an itemised list of all the substances used in the workplace or sold to clients that may be hazardous to health. Attention is drawn to any substances which may cause irritation, cause allergic reactions, burn the skin, or give off fumes.

Instructions for handling and disposing of all hazardous substances must be made available to all staff and training provided, if required. Manufacturers will usually supply information relating to their products and therapists should be able to recognise hazard warning symbols on labels and packaging.

Manual Handling Operations Regulations 1992

This legislation covers musculoskeletal disorders primarily caused by manual handling and lifting, repetitive strain disorders and unsuitable posture causing back pain. The regulations under this legislation covers minimising risks from lifting and handling large or heavy objects and require certain measures to be taken such as correct lifting techniques to avoid musculoskeletal disorders.

Fire Precautions Act 1971

This legislation is concerned with fire prevention and adequate means of escape in the event of a fire. The act enforces that:

- all premises have fire fighting equipment that is in good working order
- that the equipment is readily available and is suitable for all types of fire
- all staff are familiar with the establishments evacuation procedures and the use of fire-fighting equipment
- fire escapes are kept free from obstruction and clearly signposted
- smoke alarms are fitted
- fire doors are fitted to help control the spread of fire

It is a legal requirement for an employer to apply for a fire certificate if the business employs twenty of more staff.

It is important for all establishments to have set procedures in the event of a fire and that all staff are aware of it.

FIRE EXTINGUISHERS

There are different fire extinguishers designed to deal with different types of fire.

From 1997, all fire extinguishers must be coloured red, but they all have different symbols and colour codes to show what type of fire they should be used for.

The main types of fire extinguishers are as follows;
■ Water (Red)
■ CO_2 (Black)
■ Dry Powder (Blue)
■ Foam (Cream)

The above fire extinguishers are coded in order to allow quick and easy identification and to avoid using the wrong type and put yourself and others in danger.

The main body colour of the extinguisher has changed over the past few years (any new extinguisher purchased or leased will be predominately red), however the type colour have remained the same.

NB. Any extinguishers that are not of the correct colour will be replaced when they become unserviceable.

Water extinguishers are usually colour coded Red.

Other types of extinguishers fall into different categories, either:
■ the entire body of the extinguisher is coloured in the type colour
■ predominately red with a 5% second colour to indicate the contents of the extinguisher
■ predominately red with a bold coloured block in the relevant colour stating its type

If you are in any doubt about the type of fire extinguisher to use in the workplace, it is advisable to contact your local Fire Safety Department for advice.

Health & Safety (First Aid) Regulation 1981

Under the Health and Safety (First-Aid) Regulations 1981 workplaces must have first-aid provision. The form it should take will depend on various factors including the nature and degree of hazards at work, what medical services are available and the number of employees. The HSE booklet **COP 42 FIRST AID AT WORK (ISBN 0 11 885536 0)** contains an Approved Code of Practice and guidance notes to help employers meet their obligations.

The number of first-aiders needed in the workplace depends primarily on the degree of hazards. If the workplace is considered to be low-hazard (such as a holistic therapy clinic) there should be at least one first aider for very 50 employees.

If there are fewer than 50 employees, there should always be an appointed person present when people are at work if no trained first-aider is available.

First aiders must undertake training and obtain qualifications approved by the HSE. At present, first aid certificates are valid for three years. Refresher courses should be started before a certificate expires, otherwise a full course will need to be taken.

First Aid Kits

First aid kits should only contain items that a first-aider has been trained to use. They should always be adequately stocked and should **NOT** contain medication of any kind.

A general purpose first aid kit will contain the following items: bandages, plasters, wound dressings, antiseptic cream, quick sling, eye pads, scissors, safety pins and vinyl gloves.

First aiders should record all cases they treat. Each record should include at least the name of the patient, date, place, time and circumstances of the accident and details of the injury and treatment given.

Emergency Procedures

In the event of an emergency in the workplace (fire, accident etc) it is important to remain calm and act quickly
- Dial 999 and ask for the relevant service
- Speak clearly giving details of the emergency
- Listen carefully to any instructions you are given

Reporting of Injuries, Diseases and Dangerous Occurrences Regulations 1985 (RIDDOR)

This Legislation requires that all accidents which occur in the workplace, however minor **MUST** be entered into an accident register. This is a requirement of the Health and Safety at Work Act.

An accident report form should detail the following information:
- details of the injured person (age, sex, occupation and contact details)
- date and time of the accident
- place where the accident occurred
- a brief description of the accident
- the nature of the injury
- the action taken
- signatures of all parties concerned (preferable)

The regulations under this legislation also require that if anyone is seriously injured or dies in connection with an accident in the workplace, or if anyone is off work for more than 3 days as a result of an accident at work, or if a specified occupational disease is certified by a doctor, then the employer must send a report to the Local Authority Environmental Health Department within seven days.

DEALING WITH SPILLAGES, BREAKAGES AND WASTE IN THE WORKPLACE

When handling a **SPILLAGE**:
- wipe up immediately and warn staff and clientele. If the area is still wet display a sign indicating the potential hazard

When handling **BREAKAGES**
- clear up immediately
- wrap up sharp items such as glass before placing them into the waste refuse

When handling **WASTE**
- dispose of in a covered bin
- remove daily

Safety and Security in the Workplace

The proprietor of a Salon or Clinic is required by law to ensure adequate security of their business premises. The following steps may be taken to ensure maximum security. This is important not only for peace of mind for also for insurance requirements. Security Recommendations include:
- fitting locks and bolts on doors and windows
- installing a burglar alarm
- fitting security lights
- ensuring there are a minimum number of key holders
- leaving a light on at night, preferably at the front of the premises
- ensuring all windows and doors are checked before leaving the premises

Money
- have a safe for short-term storage of money and valuables
- always keep the till locked with a minimum number of key holders
- never leave money in the till overnight

Stock

A good stock control system is needed in the workplace in order to monitor the use of consumables and retail products and this should be documented in a stock control book. Recommendations for safeguarding stock include:

- always keeping supplies in a locked cupboard
- issuing keys to a limited number of authorised staff only
- have a locked cabinet for display purposes or use a 'dummy stock' to avoid shoplifting

Personal Belongings

It is not possible for therapists to take responsibility for a client's personal belongings when they attend for treatments. It is important for clients to be aware of this by displaying a disclaimer sign in a reception area.

When clients are removing jewellery, it is important for valuable items to be placed in a safe place for the duration of the treatment. In order to minimise risks, it is advisable to recommend that clients keep a minimum amount of money and valuables on them. Staff should be vigilant over their own property as well as that of clients and keep handbags and other items of value in a safe place.

Employers Liability Act 1969

This legislation requires the employer to provide insurance cover against claims for injury or illness as a result of negligence by the employer or other employees.

A certificate of Employers Liability insurance must be displayed in the workplace.

Local Authority Bye-Laws

Local Authorities may have their own legislation and local laws in relation to the salons and clinics providing treatments. However, the position is not uniform and will vary from County to County. It is therefore wise to seek the advice of the Local Authority Environmental Health Officer. It is worth remembering that the Trading Standards and Environmental Health Departments at the Local Authority office will have a variety of leaflets and resources relating to Legislation and these may be updated from time to time.

Consumer Legislation

It is important for therapists to be aware of the implications of Consumer Legislation in the unfortunate event of having to deal with a client seeking compensation for products or services received. Clients have a right to expect quality in respect to the service they receive, the products used on them during a treatment and products sold to them for home use.

Consumer Legislation is designed to protect any person who buys goods or services to ensure that:

- the goods are of mechandable quality
- the goods are not faulty
- there is an accurate description of the good or service

The Sale of Goods Act 1979/The Supply of Goods and Services Act 1982

As consumers of products and services, clients do have rights under the Sale of Goods Act 1979 and the Supply of Goods and Services Act 1982. This legislation identifies the contract of sale, which takes place between the retailer (the clinic/salon) and the consumer (the client).

The Sale of Goods Act 1979 was the first of the laws and covers rights including the goods being accurately described without misleading the consumer. The Supply of Goods and Services Act 1982 covers rights relating to the standards of service, in that goods and services provided should be of reasonable mechandable quality, described accurately, and be fit for their intended purpose. The act also requires that the service provided to a consumer should be carried out with reasonable skill and care, within a reasonable time and for a reasonable cost.

The Sale and Supply of Goods Act 1994

This legislation amends the previous Acts and has introduced guidelines on defining the quality of goods.

Consumer Protection Act 1987

This Act provides the consumer with protection when buying goods or services to ensure that products are safe for use on the client during the treatment, or are safe to be sold as a retail product. The Act provides the same rights to anyone injured by a defective product, where the product was sold to them or not.

The Act also covers giving misleading price indications about goods, services or facilities. The term price indication also includes price comparisons. To be misleading includes any wrongful indications about conditions attached to a price, about what you expect to happen to a price in the future and what you say in price comparisons.

It is essential to understand the implications of this legislation, including the promotion of special offers as an offence could result in legal proceedings.

Trade Descriptions Act 1968 (amended 1987)

This Act prohibits the use of false descriptions or to sell or offer the sale of goods that have been described falsely. This Act covers advertisements such as oral descriptions, display cards and applies to quality and quantity as well as fitness for purpose and price.

It is important to understand its provision, where the description is given by another person and repeated. Thus to repeat a manufacturers claim is to be equally liable.

Data Protection Act 1984

This legislation protects clients' personal information being stored on a computer.

If client records are stored on computer, the establishment must be registered under this Act.

The Data Protection Act operates to ensure that the information stored is only used for the purposes for which it was given. Businesses should therefore ensure that they:
- only hold information which is relevant
- allow individuals access to the information held on them
- prevent unauthorised access to the information

Performing Rights Act

If a therapist is using relaxation music when carrying out treatments in the workplace it may be necessary to obtain a licence from Phonographic Performance Ltd (PPL) or the Performing Rights Society (PRS) which is a organisation that collects licence payments as royalties on behalf of performers and record companies, whose music is protected under the Copyright Designs and Patent Act 1998.

When seeking to play music in treatment premises it is important to check whether the music is 'copyright free', in which case no licence fee is due, or whether it is protected under this legislation.

Maintaining Operations and Services

The role of a therapist in the context of the workplace is not merely in the provision of treatments, but in monitoring and maintaining the operations to meet the requirements of both the establishment and the client.

There are several important factors to be taken account of when working as a therapist in order to monitor and maintain the standard of service offered to clients.

It is not only important to be able to perform a skill such as Indian Head Massage competently but to be able to apply it in a way in which it is commercially acceptable.

Establishment Rules

A therapist should understand that their work activities and responsibilities must comply with the individual establishment rules in which they are working.

Establishment rules lay down a benchmark of standards required by the workplace and are set according to the requirements of the individual business.

In the workplace, therapists have a responsibility to their manager or supervisor, to their clients and to their colleagues.

THE RESPONSIBILITIES OF A THERAPIST TO A SUPERVISOR is to ensure that they:

- adhere to the establishments rules
- understand and adhere to legislation in relation to the provision of services
- report any hazard or potential danger observed in the workplace
- have a sincere commitment to provide a high standard of work to enhance the reputation and image of the establishment
- carry out work practices with honesty and integrity
- complete records fully and accurately
- are working within their own initiative to make the best use of time at work
- provide a high standard of work to ensure client satisfaction and repeat business
- create a good working relationship with other colleagues to enhance a good working environment
- avoid wastage of resources
- make recommendations for improvement in workplace practices, where appropriate
- understand how their job role contributes to the success of the business

THE RESPONSIBILITIES OF A THERAPIST TO A CLIENT ARE TO:

- treat clients with dignity and respect
- respond to clients requests politely and efficiently
- accurately inform them of the services provided by the establishment
- provide treatment only when there is a reasonable expectation that it will be advantageous to the client
- take appropriate measures to protect the client's right to privacy and confidentiality
- provide a high standard of service to ensure client satisfaction and the fostering of repeat business
- make recommendations for future treatments that would benefit the client
- make recommendations for home care products that may enhance their condition

THE RESPONSIBILITIES OF A THERAPIST TO THEIR COLLEAGUES ARE TO:
- create a good working environment by being friendly, helpful and approachable
- share responsibilities fairly to enhance a good team spirit
- ensure good communication channels pass on messages promptly and record messages accurately
- informing others of any changes in establishment procedure

Maintaining Effective Relationships with Colleagues

A successful business depends on a good image and reputation, but also depends on the way in which staff work together as a team to maintain the image and professionalism of the establishment.

Working with colleagues as a team helps enhance smooth operations and promotes a pleasant working environment and a friendly atmosphere. Working as a team involves:
- building a good rapport with each other
- understanding each other responsibilities
- working efficiently within your own job responsibilities
- responding to each others requests politely and co-operatively
- providing support and assistance, when required
- working together for the needs of the business

Communication is essential when working with others in a team, regular meetings can help to maintain effective working relationships. Meetings provide an opportunity to:
- identify and resolve problems in the workplace
- avoid breakdown in communication and misunderstandings
- contribute and exchange ideas on how workplace practices may be enhanced
- identify training needs
- maintain good working relationships

Communication skills

Whether a small or a large business, a successful business relies on good communication. Communication skills are extremely important when there are several colleagues working together and if communication is broken down, it can have a dramatic effect on the service given and the overall efficiency and image of the establishment.

It is therefore important for a therapist to be able to communicate effectively with clients, colleagues and other visitors who may visit or telephone the establishment.

Communication skills may be used to:
- identify client's needs
- inform clients about a service
- inform clients and colleagues of changes in procedures
- maintain workplace records

Communication skills involve verbal communication, listening, non-verbal communication and written communication.

VERBAL COMMUNICATION – this involves sending and receiving information and is co-operative effort between two parties. In order to facilitate effective verbal communication it is important to pause periodically in order to verify the message received was the message intended. In this way, alternations and corrections to the conversation may be made.

The objective of verbal communication is to be heard *and* understood. For clarity, it is important to choose words which convey intent clearly, concisely and tactfully.

LISTENING – although it is important to facilitate effective verbal communication, it is equally important to have good listening skills in order to develop optimal client-therapist/client-colleague relationships. Effective listening involves understanding and evaluating the person's needs, including the tone and emotion in which the message is delivered. The objective of listening is focussing on understanding the message heard.

Good communication may be enhanced by maintaining eye contact, nodding, using verbal phrases or facial expression in order to encourage the speaker to continue.

When listening it is important for therapists to clarify information received from clients or colleagues in order to ensure you understood the message correctly.

NON-VERBAL COMMUNICATION – this involves messages transmitted other than by the spoken word and may be exhibited by posture, gestures and facial expressions. Non-verbal communication often projects more information about how a person is feeling and their emotions.

As a therapist's role is in dealing with people, it is helpful to be aware of body language as this may have more meaning than the spoken word.

WRITTEN COMMUNICATION – an efficient working environment providing services to clients relies on accurate, legible record keeping, which is kept up to date. Records may either be computer based or hand written. Written communication may involve the recording of messages to colleagues to ensure continuity of service, or the completion of client records in the workplace to ensure therapeutic continuity.

In the workplace, it is very important that all messages are should be recorded accurately to ensure continuity of operation and services. Written communication should be clear, dated and timed, along with the action required. It should also be placed where the person it is intended for will notice it. Client records should be completely fully, accurately and legibly at the time of the treatment.

RESPONDING TO CLIENT'S REQUESTS

As clients are at the centre of every business it is essential for therapists to respond to their requests promptly, accurately and enthusiastically. Requests for information may come from a telephone enquiry, a personal caller to the workplace or may be in the form of a written request.

It is important to assume a friendly and approachable manner when dealing with clients requests and use phrases such as 'how may I help you'? It is also important to provide accurate information on treatments such as:

- the benefits of the services
- the cost (of individual and courses of treatment)
- the treatment duration
- any pre-treatment advice
- how often the client should attend for maximum benefit

Providing as much useful information at the time of request will increase the chances of the client booking an appointment and even if the client does not book immediately, it will certainly give them a good impression of the professionalism of the establishment.

The best source of information should be from the professionals themselves (the therapist), however, when this is not possible it is important to consider that leaflets and brochures may also help to sell treatments to clients. The information contained within leaflets and brochures should therefore be educational and informative to increase client awareness of the treatment as well as being attractive enough to stimulate interest.

Quality Assurance

Every business, however small should have a quality assurance policy in order to ensure their services and operation is conducted in a systematic way. Quality assurance policies help to monitor the quality and standard of the service provided and are useful in analysing whether the client's needs are met efficiently, effectively and consistently. Effective ways of monitoring quality assurance include:

- examining your own workplace practice and how it relates to client needs and the needs of the business
- ensuring that you don't become complacent and continue updating your skills and knowledge
- distributing client satisfaction questionnaires
- introducing a client suggestions box
- implementing changes based on recommendations from clients and staff

Encouraging communication with clients on a regular basis can help to monitor the quality assurance policy of the establishment.

Efficient work practices – cost-effectiveness

Efficient work practice requires a therapist to perform a skill to the required standard of the establishment and the Industry, and in a time which is considered to be commercially acceptable.

Cost-effectiveness in terms of the workplace means maintaining treatment times and minimising waste in order to avoid loss of revenue for the establishment. Therapists need to be aware that by adhering to their appointment times and avoiding wastage they are in fact help to preserve the business's precious resources and are thereby helping to maintain their security of employment.

Self Assessment Questions

1. Describe 3 ways in which a therapist practising Indian Head Massage may ensure that their work activities meet health and safety requirements

2. State 3 hygiene considerations which should be carried out when practising Indian Head Massage

3. What are the responsibilities of an employer under the Health and Safety and Work Act 1974?

4. Explain the significance of the following type of Legislation to a therapist:

a) Control of Substances Hazardous to Health (COSHH) 1998

b) Fire Precautions Act 1971

c) Health and Safety (First Aid Regulations 1981)

5. Which Legislation is concerned with the following in the workplace:

a) All electrical equipment being checked regularly?

b) Risks associated with manual handling and lifting?

c) The reporting of accidents?

d) Protecting clients' personal information being stored on a computer?

e) The prohibition of goods and/or services being offered for sale that have been described falsely?

6. Explain the importance of good communication skills in the workplace

7. State 3 ways in which a therapist can help to enhance workplace operations and services

8. Explain the importance of the term cost effectiveness in the workplace

CHAPTER 6

Stress Management

Stress is a common feature of modern life and is therefore something everyone experiences. Nobody is born knowing how to handle stress and as there is no immunity from it; the best way to protect the body from the harmful effects of stress is to learn how to manage it.

Stress undermines the state of physical and emotional well being; learning how to manage stress effectively can therefore help to maintain good health and vitality.

It is now acknowledged that many medical conditions are stress-related and therefore more importance is being placed on being able to handle stress in order to improve health.

The increase in stress levels is a major factor responsible for the increase in popularity of holistic therapies such as Indian Head Massage, as the value of stress relief and relaxation provided by treatments can be a major factor in helping clients to manage their own stress.

By the end of this chapter you will be able to relate the following to your work in Indian Head Massage:

- Definition of stress
- Different types of stress and how they affect the body
- Recognising stress
- Strategies to help clients to take control of and manage their own stress.
- Indian Head Massage as a counterbalance to stress

By the very nature of their work, holistic therapists are exposed to a considerable amount of emotional energy when dealing with clients. It is therefore important for them to be able to use stress management techniques in order to help both their clients and themselves.

Indian Head Massage can be a very effective treatment in counterbalancing some of the negative effects of stress, however for long term stress relief clients often need to consider many other factors in their life. This chapter considers the basics tools of stress management from identifying the symptoms and causes to employing strategies for coping with stress.

DEFINITION OF STRESS

There is no conclusive definition to the word stress. It is a difficult term to define, as stress means different things to different people.

However, it can be said that stress is the adaptive response to the demands or pressures placed upon an individual, and can involve any interference that disturbs a person's emotional and physical well being. The stress becomes unacceptable when the pressures are beyond the control of the individual and the results of the stress can then be harmful to others. Stress is therefore the imbalance between the demands of everyday life and the ability to cope.

Stress can be positive in that it can act as a stimulus and increases levels of alertness, but can also be negative when too much stress affects the ability to function effectively. It is the depth and number of stressors at any time that causes stress to become beyond control which then requires the body to make adjustments to re-establish a normal balance.

TYPES OF STRESS

Survival Stress

This type of stress is when the body reacts to meet the demands of a physically or emotionally threatening situation. The reaction is mediated by the release of adrenaline and produces the so-called 'fight or flight' reaction.

This type of stress is positive in that it enables the body and mind to react quickly and effectively. It is only when the effects of adrenaline are long term that it can lead to negative stress.

Internally Generated Stress

This type of stress is often caused by the view or reaction to a situation, rather than the situation itself. Anxiety and worry can lead to negative thought processes and often lead to a feeling that circumstances are out of control.

There is a relationship between personality and stress, in particular with anxious and obsessional personalities. What may be stressful for one person may be enjoyable and exciting for another.

Work/Lifestyle-related Stress

Many stresses that are experienced may relate to work or lifestyle. In this context, stress may come from some of following:
- having too much or too little work
- time pressures and deadlines

- demands of a job with limited resources
- insufficient working or living space
- disorganised working conditions
- limited time to the detriment of leisure and family life
- pollution
- financial problems
- relationship problems
- ill health
- family situations such as a birth, death, marriage or divorce

Negative Stress

This type of stress is caused by the inability to manage long term stress.

HOW TO RECOGNISE STRESS

Recognising stress can be very difficult. It is important to realise that as stress levels increase, the ability to recognise stress usually decreases. Stress can manifest itself in different ways, and symptoms may be presented in a number of different ways. These are discussed below.

Short Term Physical Stress Signals

These are symptoms of survival stress as the body adapts to situations that are perceived as a threat. Effects of short term physical stress include an increased heart beat, rapid breathing, increased sweating, tense muscles, dry mouth, frequency of urination, feeling of nausea.

Whilst the effects of short term physical stress may help you survive in a threatening situation, it can become negative stress when the adrenaline is not put to this use.

The effects of excess adrenaline can lead to anxiety, frustration, negative thinking, reduction in self-confidence, distraction, and may cause difficult situations to be seen as a threat rather than a challenge.

Long Term Stress Signals

Common complaints relating to long-term stress are back pain, headaches, aches and pains, excessive tiredness, digestive problems, frequent colds, skin eruptions and exacerbation of asthma. Stress and pressure can also lead to the following:

a) **INTERNAL STRESS SIGNALS**

When the body is subjected to long term stress, the mind becomes unable to think clearly and rationally about situations and problems. This can lead to feelings of anxiety, worry, confusion, feeling out of control or overwhelmed, restlessness, frustration, irritability, hostility, impatience, helplessness, depression and mood changes.

People who suffer from long term stress may generally feel more lethargic, find difficulty sleeping, change their eating habits, rely more on medication, drink and smoke more frequently and have a reduced sex drive.

b) BEHAVIOURAL STRESS SIGNALS

When people are under pressure this can be exhibited in some of the following ways: talking too fast, twitching and fiddling, being irritable, defensive, aggressive, irritated, critical and may overreact emotionally to situations. They may also find that they start becoming more forgetful, make more mistakes, are unable to concentrate, unrealistic in their judgement and become unreasonably negative. Pressure may cause some people to neglect their personal appearance and have increasing amounts of time absent from work.

If the body is subjected to excessive short term stress, it may lead to ineffective performance which should be treated as a warning sign; stress management strategies can be adopted to avoid the problem in the future. The effects of long term stress, however, can be much more severe as it can lead to extreme fatigue, exhaustion, burn-out or even breakdown.

Summary of Signs and Symptoms of Stress

1) BEHAVIOURAL CHANGES
People who suffer from stress may:
- be argumentative
- be less friendly
- become withdrawn
- avoid friends and relatives
- lose creativity
- work longer and harder and achieve less
- be reluctant to do their own job properly
- procrastinate

2) CHANGE OF FEELINGS:
People who experience stress may:
- lose their of sense of humour
- have a sense of being a failure
- lack self-esteem and have a cynical and bitter attitude
- experience irritability with conflict at home and work
- feel apathetic

3) CHANGE OF THINKING

Stress can cause people to:

- be rigid in their thinking with resistance to change
- be suspicious
- have poor concentration
- feel like leaving a job or relationship

4) PHYSICAL

People who are stressed may:

- feel tired all the time
- experience sleep problems (usually poor sleep)
- be increasingly absent from work due to prolonged minor illnesses
- have aches and pains
- suffer backache
- experience headaches and migraine
- have indigestion
- hyperventilate
- have palpitations

5) MENTAL HEALTH

The effects of stress can cause feelings of:

- anxiety
- depression
- fear of rejection

6) COGNITIVE DISTORTION

Individuals suffering from stress may view themselves in a distorted way:

- **JUMPING TO CONCLUSIONS**: even in the absence of proof, stressed individuals may jump to conclusions. They may assume that other people see them in a certain way, or they may anticipate that things will turn out badly and act as if their predictions are facts.
- **ALL OR NONE**: this is the feeling that, if you fail in one way, you see yourself as a total failure. There is then the tendency to overgeneralise to see this single failure as a proof of your life's failure.
- **MENTAL FILTER**: this is when people pick out negative events and dwell on them to the exclusion of everything else. Eventually the positive aspects of life become rejected and ignored.

THE EFFECTS OF STRESS ON THE BODY

When the body is placed under physical or psychological stress, it increases the production of certain hormones such as cortisol and adrenaline. These hormones produce marked changes in the heart rate, blood pressure levels, metabolism and physical activity. Whilst this physical action can help a person to function more effectively when under pressure for short periods of time, it can also be extremely damaging and debilitating in the long term.

Dr Hans Selye called the body's response to stress the 'general adaptation syndrome' which he suggested be divided into 3 stages.

The first stage is the **ALARM STAGE** which is the body's initial reaction to the perceived stressor. This involves the so-called fight or flight syndrome which involves the sympathetic nervous system and the release of the hormones adrenaline and cortisol.

The effects on the body are to effect an alert response, and include:

■ increased heart rate
■ increased ventilation rate
■ increased diversion of blood to the muscles and brain
■ increase in perspiration
■ increased release of glucose from the liver
■ inhibited digestion

The alarm stage allows the body to cope and respond and when the threat is over the body returns to a state of balance through repair and rest (parasympathetic system)

However, problems can start to occur when the restoration of balance does not occur through not allowing the body to rest sufficiently, or through perceived or real encounters with repeated stressful situations.

Repeated alarm reactions can lead to symptoms such as breathlessness, a dry mouth, aching, a clenched jaw or fists, dizziness, palpitations and sweating.

The second stage is known as the resistance stage, which through the secretion of the circulating hormones allows the body to continue fighting long after the effects of the alarm reaction have dissipated. This eventually leads to symptoms of disease as the body's energy resources are drained without adequate recuperation and repair. Symptoms associated with the resistance stage include colds and flu, anxiety and depression, high blood pressure, chest pains, tiredness, insomnia, indigestion, headaches and migraine.

The third stage is the exhaustion stage which takes place if the stress response continues without relief and can result in organs becoming more and more compromised until the adaptation becomes degenerative.

> **KEY NOTE** Increased cortisol secretion in stressful situations reduces the body's immune response and the anti-inflammatory effect of cortisol can slow down healing too.

Areas of the Body Most Vulnerable to Stress

When the body is moving or stationary, a combination of muscle tension and relaxation exists in order to maintain posture.

If a good balance is not achieved then the body suffers excessive muscle tension which can cause pain and fatigue. If muscles are held tightly in a state of contraction, circulation is impeded which results in a buildup of the products of fatigue. This can then result in muscular spasms, aches and pains.

When under stress, the entire body becomes tense and posture changes. Hours spent sitting and working at a desk can cause tension to accumulate in the upper body, particularly around the neck and shoulders. Large amounts of time spent in front of the computer screen can result in eyestrain where the eyes and surrounding muscles become tired.

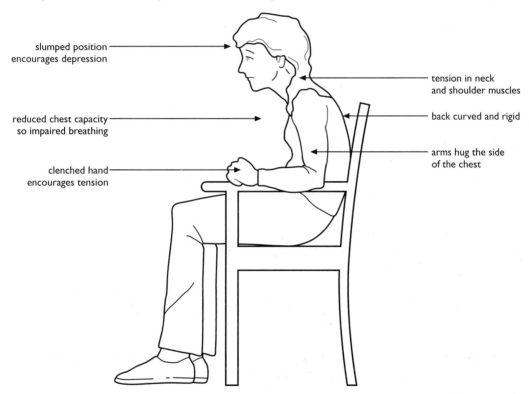

slumped position encourages depression

reduced chest capacity so impaired breathing

clenched hand encourages tension

tension in neck and shoulder muscles

back curved and rigid

arms hug the side of the chest

Being tense and in a permanent state of alert can be uncomfortable and has the ability to throw the body out of balance. Tension uses up energy, but the energy is unproductive. Muscle tension can also affect the ability to function well as it makes our thought processes less efficient.

> **KEY NOTE** Tension can also have a debilitating effect on the immune system, predisposing people to colds and other diseases, as when in a constant state of alert, it inhibits healing and tissue repair. The key to stress relief is therefore relaxation as healing can only take place when the body is at rest.

The Shoulders

The shoulders are the place where most people hold a considerable amount of tension. When the body in a state of tension the shoulders are lifted towards the ears and often remain this way causing the muscles to go into spasm. This restricts the blood flow to the head, neck and shoulders and causes the neck and shoulders to become stiff and inflexible. Sitting with hunched shoulders can reduce chest capacity and thus impair breathing.

> **KEY NOTE** Indian Head Massage can help to counterbalance the effects of stress, as by relaxing the shoulders they will drop and allow the energy to flow more freely to the area, encouraging deeper and easier breathing and improved joint flexibility.

Upper Arms

The upper arms are important for upper body movement and when the shoulders are tense they tighten and restrict movement.

When in a state of tension, the upper arms tend to hug the chest either at the sides or in front, whilst the elbows bend up.

> **KEY NOTE** Indian Head Massage can help to reduce tension and tightness in the upper arm muscles to help improve flexibility of the arms and shoulders.

Neck

When the body is balanced the neck is designed allow the head to move in a variety of directions. When the body is out of balance and under stress, the head tends to come forwards and the chin juts out. This then throws the body out of alignment as the neck muscles tense and take the weight of the head. The neck muscles are then in a permanent state of contraction and can cause the neck to become stiff and tight. The tension then reduces mobility of the neck and shoulders.

> **KEY NOTE** Working on the neck with Indian Head Massage helps to open up the energy flow from the spine to the whole head and can help to reduce tension, improve posture by re-aligning the muscles, thereby increasing mobility and-allowing the head to move more freely.

Head

The face is an area of the body that cannot help but show tension; the jaw clamps tight, teeth grind together and the lips tighten. The scalp muscles, along with the temporal muscles tighten when under stress restricting the blood flow, leading to headaches, eyestrain and neck and shoulder tension.

> **KEY NOTE** Indian Head Massage helps to counterbalance stress in the head by improving the circulation, relaxing the muscles and nerve fibres, thereby relieving tension.

When the body is in balance it facilitates relaxation and a positive mental outlook, which is critical to successful stress management.

If the shoulders and chest are free of tension the ribs are free to allow deep relaxed breathing; if the head and neck are well balanced they can support the shoulders and take pressure from the neck muscles.

The body is ideally equipped to deal with many different types of stressors, however the ability to deal with stress can be inhibited by a heavy load of unresolved stress, which contributes to the development of disease and pain.

STRESS RELATED DISORDERS

Stress is considered to be a contributory factor in many conditions. Listed below are areas susceptible to stress-related diseases:

SKIN – as the skin is often a manifestation of what is felt inside disorders; skin disorders such as eczema and psoriasis are often exacerbated by stress. Allergies may also be triggered by stress.

HAIR – some forms of hair loss are linked to stress.

HEART – high blood pressure and conditions such as angina may be exacerbated by stress. If the blood supply to the heart is restricted by arteriosclerosis and the person's life is very stressful a heart attack can result.

LUNGS – symptoms of asthma often worsen when the body is subjected to high levels of emotional stress.

MUSCLES – muscle tension is often the result of stress.

BRAIN – anxiety and depression may be triggered by stress.

REPRODUCTIVE – the reproductive hormones are reduced at times of stress; this is evidenced by stress-related problems such as infertility and menstrual disorders.

DIGESTION – conditions that may be aggravated by stress include ulcers, irritable bowel syndrome.

ADAPTATION TO STRESS

Fortunately, the body has the capacity to cope with stress as the purpose of all the body's systems is to maintain a constant internal environment through homeostasis.

However there are several factors that may affect the body's ability to deal with stress which include the following:

GENETICS – the effects of stress on the body can be determined by genetic make-up and can dictate how well different organs respond and adapt to stressful situations.

PHYSIOLOGICAL RESERVE – the body's response to stress depends on the ability to increase or decrease function according to the body's needs. If the ability of the organ to respond is diminished, it is difficult for the body to maintain homeostasis; even with small demands imbalance and disease may ensue.

AGE – with age the ability to adapt is diminished and whilst a young, healthy individual may respond and adapt to stress easily, an elderly client may find the situation considerably more stressful.

HEALTH STATUS – clients who are mentally and physically fit are able to adapt to stress placed on them more easily than others who are not.

NUTRITION – deficiencies or excesses of nutrition can impair one's ability to adapt to stressful situations.

SLEEP – irregular sleep patterns and wakefulness can reduce immunity as well as physical and psychological functions. Sleep is important for restoring energy and if sleep is inadequate, it can impair the body's ability to deal with stress.

PSYCHOLOGICAL FACTORS – psychological conditions such as anxiety and depression can make a person more susceptible to stress.

MANAGING STRESS

In order to be able to work towards prevention of stress, it is firstly important to be able to identify its causes.

Part of the problem with stress is its familiarity, as people become so used to living with stress they may be unaware of how it is affecting them or those around them.

Mental attitude is a critical factor in dealing with stress, along with finding ways of reducing the effects of stress. Focusing on the ownership of the sources of the stress and not on the feelings they generate, is the first step to counterbalancing it. Stress management can be approached in several different ways and a client's stress management programme may typically consist of experiencing a range of holistic therapies, the use of relaxation and stress reduction techniques, as well as implementing lifestyle changes.

Holistic therapists can help clients to recognise their own stress by advising on ways in which they can combat it and start to manage their own stress positively. Stress Management has to take into account the recognition of an individual's vulnerability to stress, ability to be aware of possible sources of stress and identifying signs and symptoms of stress. What is most important, is helping clients to learn how to manage stress, be able to identify those factors that contribute to it and so be able to control it.

Optimum Stress Levels

Stress levels vary, like any other human characteristic and what may seem challenging and exciting to one person may seem stressful and threatening to another. The most positive approach to successful stress management is finding an optimum stress level in which the body can be sufficiently stimulated to perform well, whilst not becoming overstressed and unhappy.

> **KEY NOTE** It is important for each individual to be able to monitor their own stress levels, as some people may operate most effectively at a low level of stress, however this may leave another person feeling bored or unmotivated. Alternatively someone who performs only moderately at a low level may find they excel at a high level when they are under more pressure.

The most effective way of finding an optimum level of stress is to keep a stress diary for a short period of time, in order to be able to analyse what is causing the stress and whether it is being controlled effectively. The type of information that could be recorded in a stress diary is the stressful event and time, how stressful the event was (on a scale of 1 to 10) what made the event stressful and how the situation was handled. This can be the key to identifying whether it was the cause that was tackled or the symptom.

When analysing a stress diary, it should be possible to project the following information:
- The level of stress that is optimum for an individual
- The main sources of unpleasant or negative stress and whether the strategies for managing them are effective or not

MANAGING STRESS EFFECTIVELY

Once there is an understanding or recognition as to what is causing the stress and the level under which an individual can work effectively, the next stage is to work out how to manage the stress. An action plan for managing stress may include:
- Controlling or eliminating the problems that are causing the stress
- Using stress reduction techniques
- Making lifestyle changes
- Taking a holiday or break more often
- Social and family support
- Time management
- Hobbies and leisure time
- Being prepared to ask for help
- Looking back at action taken and evaluating the effects

Stress Reduction Techniques

When choosing methods for stress reduction, different strategies may be required for different people and different circumstances.

The main objective in managing stress is to help the client to improve the quality of their lives and their resistance to stress by employing certain techniques, as well as making certain lifestyle changes. It is important to realise that as people react differently to stress, different techniques or combination of techniques may be required for each individual.

Stress can only be eliminated if the root causes are recognised and resolved. However, there are ways in which the unpleasant effects of stress may be reduced.

Relaxation Techniques

Physical relaxation is often something which appears easy, but in practice is a skill that needs to be learnt and practised.

By teaching clients physical relaxation techniques you can help them to take responsibility for their stress reactions and reduce the distress of many conditions.

Tensing muscles and holding breath when tense becomes habitual; the key to relaxation is training the body to feel tension and recognise when breathing reflects tension.

The body's reaction to stress involves breathing and muscle tension; the parts over which a person can gain control. The aim of relaxation is to control breathing and muscle tension in order to calm the mind and body.

Through learning physical relaxation, a person can learn to slow down their breathing, breathe deeply and relax their muscles. As the relaxation response starts to happen, other responses change automatically and as the breathing calms down and the muscles relax, the heart rate simultaneously slows down. With relaxation, the key is in gaining control over breathing and muscles: the rest will happen automatically as the body responds positively to being in a state of relaxation.

Relaxation can help to:
- maintain emotional and physical health
- aid restful sleep
- reduce the harmful effects of stress
- relieve muscular tension
- promote optimum oxygen levels for the body
- actively help the body to recover and repair

Breathing

Deep breathing is a very effective method of relaxation and works well combined with other relaxation techniques such as relaxation imagery, meditation and progressive muscular relaxation.

On inhaling, the intercostal muscles, abdominal muscles and the diaphragm contract in order to increase the volume of the thoracic cavity which causes air to pass into the lungs. Whilst the breath is held, all these muscles remain tensed. When they relax, the volume of the thoracic cavity decreases as the muscles return to their original relaxed position. Comfortable, healthy breathing brings air down into the depth of the lungs and the body is able to relax as the breath is let out. When the body is still tense, breathing becomes fast and the muscles in the upper part of the chest take over to cause panting.

The experience of any physical or emotional stress will affect breathing. At times of stress, breathing becomes shallow and irregular, resulting in the brain being deprived of insufficient oxygen leading to feeling of dizziness, inability to concentrate and agitation. Learning how to breathe deeply helps to fill the body with positive energy and clears the mind. It can also help prevent a person from getting stressed, or can help them gain control more quickly when they are feeling stressed. Most people use only half of their lung capacity and breath with their chest and not their diaphragm.

Below are two breathing exercises which may be taught to clients for self-help. It is important for clients to practise breathing exercises regularly, in order that they may be prepared to use them the next time they feel anxious and stressed.

BREATHING EXERCISES FOR SUCCESSFUL STRESS CONTROL

Breathing Exercise 1

Sit in a comfortable position and loosen tight clothing.

Place one hand on the chest and the other across the stomach.

Inhale deeply through the nose to fill the upper chest cavity and down to the lower part of the lungs, as if breathing into the stomach for a count of 6.

Exhale slowly to a count of 12, allowing the air to escape from the top of your lungs first before the lower part deflates.

Repeat this exercise 6-8 times

Breathing Exercise 2

Apply the first two fingers of the right hand to the side of the right nostril and press gently to close it. Breathe in slowly through the left nostril and hold for a count of 3.

Transfer the first two fingers to the left nostril to close it.

Breathe out slowly through the right nostril on a count of 3. Breathe in through the right nostril and hold for a count of 3 and whilst holding transfer the fingers to the right nostril and breathe out.

Repeat the exercise 6 times

NOTE After completing breathing exercises clients should be advised to wait a few moments before getting up to avoid dizziness.

Correct breathing is something which really needs to be practised often until it feels natural and it may be then be utilised as a counterbalance to stress. Breathing properly enables the body to relax and regain its natural balance, whilst calming the mind. If a client has difficulty breathing correctly, it may be advisable for them to attend classes which involve structured breathing such as yoga.

The effects of poor breathing on the body can be damaging in that it:
- weakens the nervous system
- encourages muscle tension
- starves the body of nutrients
- blocks the circulation
- weakens the immune system
- disturbs digestion

Progressive Muscular Relaxation

This is a physical technique, designed to relax the body when it is tense. It may be applied to any group of muscles in the body, depending on whether one area is tense of whether it is the whole body.

PMR is achieved by tensing a group of muscles so that they are as tightly contracted as possible. The muscles are then held in a state of tension for a few seconds and relaxed. This should result in a feeling of deep relaxation in the muscles.

For maximum effect, this exercise should be combined with breathing exercises and imagery (such as the image of stress leaving the body).

Relaxation Exercise

Find a place where you can feel comfortable.

Close your eyes and pull your feet towards you as far as you can, hold them for a count of 5 and let them relax. Let them drop as if you are a puppet on a string and the string has broken.

Curl your toes as if you were holding a pencil, hold them for a count of 5 and then relax.

Tighten and tense the calf muscles, count to 5 and then relax.

Tighten and tense the thighs, press then tightly together, count to 5 and then relax allowing them to fall apart.

Tighten the abdominal muscles, pulling in the muscles, count to 5 and then relax.

Tighten the muscles in the hips and the buttocks, count to 5 and then relax.

Arch the back and tense the back muscles, count to 5 and then relax.

Tense the shoulders by raising then to the ears, count to 5 and then drop them.

Lift your arms up with the hands outstretched as if you were reaching for something. Hold for a slow count of 5 and then let the arms drop down.

Tense the muscles in the forehead, count to 5 and then relax.

Tense the muscles around the eyes tightly, count to 5 and then relax.

Tense the muscles in the jaw and cheeks (as if gritting your teeth), hold for 5 and then relax.

By now you should feel relax and heavy, as if you are sinking into the floor or chair.

Check that all body parts are free from tension and if there are any areas left with tension, hold that part tense again before relaxing.

When you're ready get up gradually, taking your time.

NB. This exercise will be easier to do if the instructions are on tape, preferably spoken by a person with a slow, calm and relaxing voice.

Imagery and Visualisation

Imagery techniques can be useful to recreate a retreat from stress and pressure, by imagining a place or event that was happy and restful, and calling upon it to help manage a stressful period.

Imagery and visualisation is often more effective and real if it is combined with sounds, smell, taste and warmth. It is important to realise that visualisation is a very individual skill. Clients should be encouraged to call upon a happy experience, and that visualisation could be geared towards that image. Imagery and visualisation can often be enhanced by a relaxation tape which may be played while the client is receiving treatment and can be purchased for home use.

Meditation

This is a very effective way of relaxing as the idea is to focus your thoughts on relaxing for a period of time, leaving the mind and body to recover from the problems and worries that have caused the stress. Meditation can help to reduce stress by slowing down breathing, helping muscular relaxation, reducing blood pressure, help clear thinking by focusing and concentrating the mind. The key to meditation is to quieten the mind and focus completely on one thing.

With meditation, it is important for the body to be relaxed and in a comfortable position.

Meditation is a very personal experience and can involve a person sitting or laying quietly and focusing the mind, or can be taught in a class situation.

Therapists may also facilitate meditation by using positive mental imagery and visualisation in order to help clients focus their mind on their imagery and lift themselves into a state of passive awareness in order to relax.

Relaxing at Work

When spending hours sitting at a desk, driving or in meetings tension can accumulate in the areas of the body most vulnerable to stress such as the head, neck and shoulders.

Using a simple relaxation routine whilst at work can help to release tension, reduce stress and renew the body's energy to carry on working effectively.

Start by loosening any tight clothing (collar, ties, scarves) and removing your shoes

5 Minute Stress Reliever

Sit comfortably with you back supported against the back of the chair, with the feet firmly on the ground and the hand and arms open and relaxed and supported by arm rests.

1. With a deep breath in raise the shoulders towards the ears and hold them raised for a few seconds (be aware of the tension that may be accumulating in the shoulders), now take a long slow breath out and drop the shoulders down.
   Repeat this exercise several times

2. Now lift your right shoulder and slowly pop it backwards several times, ensuring that the arms and kept loose and relaxed. Repeat the exercise with the left shoulder. *Now pop both shoulders together. Repeat several times.*

3. Place your left hand on your right shoulders and squeeze gently and then release. Repeat the exercise down the right arm to the elbow. Repeat several times. Now place your right hand on your left shoulder and repeat the exercise.

4. Place your hands over your shoulders. As you exhale let your head fall backwards and slowly draw your fingers over the clavicles (collar bones). Repeat several times.

5. Place your hands over the top of your head and gently pull your head gently downwards, feeling the slight stretch in the back of the neck. Hold this position for several seconds and then repeat.

6. Place the fingers of both hands at the base of your skull apply slow circular pressures from the base of the skull and behind the ears gradually working down the neck. Repeat several times.

7. Exhale and turn the head to the right side. Hold there for a few seconds and use right hand to massage the right side of the neck from behind the eye down to the clavicle (collar bone). Repeat the exercise to the other side of the neck.

8. Now close your eyes and relax the muscles in your face, be aware of your eye muscles, your jaw and your forehead. Place the fingers of both hands on each side of the temples and slowly massage in a circular motion, repeating several times.

9. Place the fingertips of both hands in the centre of the forehead and perform slow circular movements with both hands working out towards the temples. Repeat several times.

10. Finish by cupping your hands over your eyes and holding for several seconds. This helps to release tension and tightness left in the face.

Clients can be encouraged to practise these exercises at least once a day during a break, and individual exercises may be used whenever they start to feel tense to avoid stress building up.

Stress Management is something which needs to be assessed in a holistic way, and will undoubtedly involve many other factors which include:

Welcoming Change

It is important to realise that in implementing a stress management programme, there will be an element of change, and success will often depend on the adaptation to change. Changes in circumstances and lifestyle can be stressful, however it is often the anticipation of the change that is more stressful than the change itself.

Attitude to Stress

Attitude is a fundamental factor in stress management. A negative attitude can cause stress by alienating and irritating other people whereas a positive attitude can help to draw the positive elements out of a situation and can make life more pleasurable and stress more manageable.

When the body is under stress, it is very easy to lose perspective and relatively minor problems can be perceived as threatening and intimidating. When faced with a seemingly over-whelming problem it may help to view the problem in a different way, for instance as a challenge or seeing what may be learned from it, whatever the outcome. It is important to be able to view mistakes as a learning experience and that if something has been learnt from the experience, then it has a positive value. Learning how to change the response to stress can help to transform it from a negative to a positive experience.

It may help to talk to someone who has had similar problems, or write the problem down in order to help put it into perspective. It is often helpful to break the problem down in order that it may be reduced to a smaller, more manageable size.

Positive Thinking/Cognitive Therapy

Negative thoughts can cause stress as they can damage confidence and harm effective performance by stifling rational mental thoughts. Common negative thoughts are feelings of inadequacy, self-criticism, dwelling on past mistakes and worrying about how you appear to others.

Awareness of negative thoughts can be the first step to counterbalancing stress. It is important to write negative thoughts down and review them rationally, decide whether they are based on reality. It is useful to counter negative thoughts with positive affirmations in order to change a negative thought into a positive one, such as 'I can do this'.

Stress from the Environment

Disorganised living and working conditions can be a major source of stress. A well organised and pleasant environment can usually make a large contribution to reducing stress and increasing productivity. Stress may be reduced in the environment by improving air quality, lighting, decora-tion, untidiness and noise levels. Natural light can lift moods and help prevent eyestrain. Creating order out of disorder can help clear a space mentally and physically to regain a state of calm.

When working in an office, it is advisable to consider the ergonomics of furniture as a source of potential source of stress. If working at a computer station, chairs should be checked for comfort and height and the keyboard and monitor comfortably positioned and at the right height. Taking a short break from a computer/desk work every hour or so can help prevent tension and eyestrain from building up.

HEALTH AND NUTRITION

Eating an unbalanced diet can cause stress to the body by depriving it of essential nutrients. Eating a well balanced diet can help to eliminate chemical stress that may be caused by consumption of too much caffeine, too much alcohol, smoking and eating food with high levels of sugar and salt.

Drinking more water may help to increase energy levels and the resistance to stress, by clearing the toxins from the bloodstream. By eating sensible well-balanced meals it can help to calm or energise the mind and body and counteract the effects of stress.

The best defence against negative stress is a healthy and nutritious diet.

Implementing the following guidelines with diet and nutrition can help towards successful stress control:

- taking time out to eat properly (avoid working lunches)
- eat slowly and chew food well to aid digestion
- rest for a few minutes after eating
- eat fresh food to provide the body with essential vitamins and minerals
- avoid eating late at night to allow the body time to digest food properly
- avoid overeating, as it will decrease energy levels
- avoid eating if you are feeling angry, agitated or upset (practice relaxation techniques before eating)

A healthy diet to help beat stress will consist of:

- eating food rich in vitamins such as citrus fruits and dark green leafy vegetables
- eating foods rich in vitamin A and folic acid
- cutting back on alcohol, caffeine, refined sugars, salt and saturated fats
- eating iron-rich foods such as dried beans, peas and leafy green vegetables
- eating foods high in zinc and magnesium (seafood, whole grains and dried beans)
- eating balanced amounts of protein, fat and carbohydrates to help provide the body with energy to be able to cope with stress
- eating plenty of whole, unprocessed foods (wholegrain bread and cereals, dried beans and peas, fresh fruit and vegetables, low-fat milk)
- drinking at least two pints of water a day

Exercise

Taking frequent exercise is one way of reducing stress, as it helps to improve your health, relaxes tense muscles, relaxes the mind and helps induce sleep. Exercise can help to accelerate the flow of blood through the brain, helping the brain to function more clearly, and will remove waste products that have built up as a result of intensive mental energy. Exercise also releases chemicals called endorphins into the blood stream that give a feeling of well-being.

When considering implementing exercise into a stress management programme, thought should be given to the type of exercise and its suitability to the individual, as if it is difficult or unenjoyable it may cause stress and may not be continued long enough to derive long term benefits.

Taking Time Out

A successful way of reducing long term stress is to take up a hobby where there is little or no pressure for performance. Long term stress can also be reduced by taking time out for undirected activities such as reading a book, taking a walk, having a long bath, listening to music. It is important to take regular holidays or breaks in order to refresh mind and body and recharge energy levels. Taking a break can also help to put problems into perspective.

Managing relationships (home and work)

Stress can be caused by relationships with other people and although it is not possible to change a person's personality, a change of attitude will often determine the amount of stress experienced from the situation.

A useful technique to employ when dealing with other people is to try and understand the way they think and why they feel the way they do. Unfortunately, it is human nature that people will often attempt to exploit a relationship at the expense of another person. In this case, it is important to project the right approach – by being positive, pleasant but assertive.

When dealing with a difficult, annoying or frustrating person, it is always a good policy to stay calm and neutral (take deep breaths) in order to be able to think more clearly and react more rationally. It also important to be able to respect other people's opinions and to accept that some people or situations may not change.

Indian Head Massage as an Antidote to Stress

Holistic therapies such as Indian Head Massage can help clients to manage their stress as they provide a period of time away from everyday stresses in order to relax and regain a sense of physical and emotional balance. A combination of relaxation and holistic therapy programme can relieve tension and stress and allow the body energies to flow more freely. When the body reaches a state of relaxation tense muscles start to unknot, blood pressure starts to lower, breathing becomes more regular and deeper and the mind drifts into a state of passive awareness.

Indian Head Massage is particularly effective as an antidote to stress as it relaxes and revitalises the mind and body, and can help with anxiety, tension and many stress-related conditions.

Other Professional Help

Although holistic therapies can provide a positive counterbalance to the negative effects of stress, it is important that a client does not become dependent on a therapist for any advice or service than that which is associated with the chosen treatment.

Clients may need to consult another professional, for instance if they are deeply depressed they may need to be referred to their GP or to a Counsellor.

KEY NOTE It is unhealthy for a client to become reliant on a holistic therapist for their problems and see them as the one to provide a solution to their stress.
The key to successful stress management is for clients to be able to recognise their own stress and for the therapists to help guide them as to how they may manage it.

NOTE Therapists should always take care to ensure that they remain objective with clients at all times and realise that by not taking responsibility for their problems they are in fact helping them to help themselves.

TIME MANAGEMENT

By employing time management skills effectively, time can be utilised in the most productive and effective way. Time management can help to reduce stress by increasing productivity, allowing therefore more time to relax outside of work activities.

The important factor in time management is to concentrate on results and not on activity by:
- Assessing the value of your time and how it may be used most effectively
- Focusing on priorities, whilst deciding which tasks can be delegated and which may be dropped
- Managing and avoiding distractions
- Finishing work that has been started and working systematically
- Learning when to say no and avoiding feeling guilty for saying so
- Avoiding being someone else's time problem and reducing commitments
- Having a planner for the weeks of the years, including a plan for holidays and leisure

This can help to reduce the effects of long term stress by helping to put things back into perspective, giving a feeling of control and direction and freeing more quality time to relax and enjoy life outside of work.

Evaluating Stress from Experience

In a stress management programme, it is important to look back and re-assess in order to plan for the future. Planning ahead can help you to manage stress more effectively, rather that waiting for the distress signals. It is always useful to look back on a stressful situation in order to assess whether it was dealt with successfully and in order to decide what could be repeated or what needs to be changed.

Stress Management in The Workplace

Stress is a significant factor, costing industry billions of pounds a year, as it is thought that 60% of absenteeism in the workplace is believed to be caused by stress-related disorders.

Over the last century, ever-increasing technological changes have lead to a faster pace of life and to people being required to perform the job descriptions that may previously have been assigned to several people.

Stress occurs when the body is required to perform beyond its normal range of capabilities and the net results of this can be harmful to both individuals and organisations. It is also important to realise that stress can be a motivator and that people need a certain amount of pressure in order to stimulate them into action. Positive stress is the type of stress that gives the body a kick start whenever needed. It is a known fact that people with too much time on their hands and not enough stimulus suffer from symptoms of stress, just as those do with too much and work and too little time.

Companies are starting to realise that their staff members are more productive when they are able to deal with stress creatively and any factors that can help to reduce the damaging effects of stress can make the workforce happier and increase productivity.

Part of an action plan for stress management at work may include the following:

- Learning to recognise the warning signals of stress and act on them to start taking control of stress responses
- Enlisting the support of colleagues and not being afraid to talk about stressful situations in order to relieve some of the feeling of pressure
- Taking regular breaks away from the desk or workspace and getting some fresh air (even if it means opening a window or door)
- Paying attention to the ergonomics of office furniture and trying to keep your workspace uncluttered
- Eating healthily and regularly
- Eating slowly and digesting food properly
- Learning to delegate and use time management skills – making a list and prioritising
- Keeping a stress diary, noting the days when high stress levels are experienced and learning from these to help counterbalance the negative effects in the future
- Setting realistic goals to avoid stress of failing to meet an unrealistic deadline
- Concentrating on one task at a time
- Pause after completing one task before starting another
- Planning activities for days off
- Trying to view problems as challenges and as opportunities
- Thinking positively – negative thought processes can be disabling and very destructive
- Learning to see the funny side of stressful situations
- Looking after yourself
- Using relaxation techniques regularly

Indian Head Massage as a Counterbalance to Stress in the Workplace

Many companies and individuals are now aware of the costs negative stress can have on their company and their staff. Staff illness can lead to reduced productivity, increased pressure being placed on other individuals leading to low morale and high staff turnover. Frequent complaints of work related stress include the following :

"my neck and shoulders ache constantly from using the phone all day"

"I frequently suffer from headaches at work and feel under pressure all the time to meet tight deadlines"

"I never have time for a lunch hour as there is always too much work and not enough time to complete it in"

"I feel stressed-out and tired before I even start work and am too exhausted to enjoy a social life"

Comments like those above sound all too familiar to those suffering from the negative effects of stress at work, who could benefit from stress reduction techniques.

Some organisations have occupational health advisors who look after the welfare of their staff and are interested in ways in which staff stress levels may be managed effectively. Indian Head Massage is well suited to the work environment due to its portable nature. An area of the workplace (preferably private) can be assigned for the treatment, which is performed in an ordinary chair and is short enough in duration to be slotted into a break or lunch hour. It is also advantageous in that the client does not have to undress.

The benefits of Indian Head Massage to Organisations and individuals are that it helps to:
- increase staff morale by alleviating depression and anxiety
- relieve stress and muscular tension
- relieve headaches, neck and back ache
- relieve eyestrain
- relieve mental and physical strain
- improve concentration levels, memory and mental alertness
- increase energy levels to improve productivity

Stress Management
Self Assessment Questions

1. Define the term stress

2. State 3 symptoms of:

a) Short term stress

b) Long term stress

c) Behavioural stress

3. Explain what is meant by the following in relation to the body's response to stress, as defined by Dr Hans Selye

a) The alarm stage

b) The resistance stage

c) The exhaustion stage

4. State 3 factors that affects the body's capacity to cope with stress

5. List 6 important components of an effective stress management programme

6. Describe how Indian Head Massage can be an effective antidote to stress

CHAPTER 7

Indian Head Massage Techniques

In India massage has long been adopted as a daily practice in order to help maintain a healthy mind and body throughout the course of life. In the modern day of high stress levels in the western world, massage is a must for relaxing both mind and body, and recharging depleted energy levels. Indian Head Massage is uniquely different from other types of therapeutic massage practised in the west in that it is applied through the clothes to a client in a seated position, thereby supplanting the need for special or sophisticated equipment.

By the end of this chapter you will be able to:

- Understand the massage movements used in Indian Head Massage along with their effects
- Prepare a treatment area for Indian Head Massage
- Understand the properties and benefits of oils and herbs used in Indian Head Massage
- Carry out a step-by-step Indian Head Massage treatment to the upper back and shoulders, upper arms, neck, scalp and face
- Provide after-care advice

Massage Movements used in Indian Head Massage

The massage techniques used in Indian Head Massage are simple but extremely effective. They consist of a combination of traditional Indian techniques and westernised techniques.

According to the traditional techniques of Indian Head Massage there are five main types of strokes:

1) SMOOTHING OR STROKING

These are superficial techniques applied with the whole hand, fingers or the forearms (similar to effleurage in swedish massage). Smoothing can be applied softly and gently to produce a calming effect or applied more briskly to stimulate the circulation and energise and revitalise the person being massaged.

Effects of smoothing or stroking
- dilates the capillaries and increases the circulation
- relaxes the client by soothing sensory nerve endings in the skin
- prepares the area for deeper strokes
- aids in moving waste out of congested areas
- soothes tired, achy muscles
- warms the tissues making them more extensible

2) TAPPING

These techniques are performed with the fingers and are similar to percussion and vibration movements in swedish massage. Their effects are to:
- stimulate the nerve endings
- increase the circulation and local blood flow
- waken and refresh the body

When applied lightly they are soothing and bring about relaxation and a release of tension and when applied more deeply they have a stimulating effect on the nerves and are refreshing.

3) KNEADING OR SQUEEZING

These techniques involve the thumbs or the whole hand and fingers. These movements involve the skin and muscular tissue being moved from their position and squeezed with a firm pressure away from the underlying structure and then released. Effects are:
- increases the removal of waste products from the tissue and encourages fresh oxygen and nutrients to be delivered to the tissues
- stretches muscle tissue and fascia
- reduces adhesions and muscular spasms
- relaxes muscle tissue and reduces accumulated stress and tension from the muscles

4) RUBBING OR FRICTIONS

A strong feature of the Indian Head Massage are the deep friction movements which are performed with the whole of the hand, the heel of the hand or the fingers, and the lighter technique of rubbing using the ball and the heel of the hand. Rubbing excites the circulation and increases heat in the area being massaged because of the friction. Effects of Rubbing or Frictions are to:

- dilate the capillaries and increase the circulation
- generate heat
- loosen stiffness and tension by relaxing muscles
- break down and help free adhered tissue in restricted areas

5) PRESSURES

These movements are applied with the fingers and the thumbs and their general effects are to:

- clear congestion in the nerve pathways
- increase circulation
- restore energy balance to the body

EQUIPMENT AND MATERIALS FOR INDIAN HEAD MASSAGE

The beauty of Indian Head Massage lies in its simplicity. It can be performed in an ordinary chair, without the need to purchase expensive equipment.

> - The type of chair best suited to Indian head Massage treatments is one with a relatively low back and without an arm rest.
> - An important factor for the therapist is the height of the chair; it is therefore preferable for the therapist to work with a chair with an adjustable height and back rest to ensure correct body mechanics.

It is also important for a therapist practising Indian Head Massage to have a variety of oils for optional use on the scalp and a hand cleanser. The type of hand cleanser most suited to a visiting therapist are dry anti-bacterial cleansers which are easy and practical to use.

OILS USED IN INDIAN HEAD MASSAGE

The use of oil is optional when massaging the scalp. Oil that is applied to the head is absorbed into the roots of the hair which are connected with nerve fibres leading to the brain.

Applying oil to the head helps to strengthen the hair, remove dryness, and by relaxing the muscles and nerves of the head, fatigue is eliminated leaving the recipient feeling refreshed and revitalised.

Massaging the head increases a fresh supply of oxygen and glucose to the brain and improves the circulation of spinal fluid around the brain and the spinal cord.

There are several oils which may be used for Indian Head Massage.

Traditionally oils such as sesame, coconut, olive, mustard and almond have been used by Indian women as part of their grooming ritual to keep their hair in good condition.

> **KEY NOTE** When the body is subjected to stress and illness, the skin and hair are often affected resulting in dryness and sometimes loss of hair.
> With tension the scalp becomes tight, restricting the flow of nutrients to the hair to promote healthy hair growth.
> Using oils on a regular basis can help to encourage healthy shiny hair, slow down hair loss and soften and moisturise the hair.

ALMOND OIL – being high in nutrients such as unsaturated fatty acids, protein and vitamins A, B, D & E, this oil makes an excellent hair conditioner, helping to soften, moisturise and protect the hair. It has warming effects on the body and is therefore useful for stimulating hair growth, as well as helping to reduce muscular pain and tightness.

COCONUT OIL – this is a popular oil for Indian Head Massage and is widely used in southern parts of India. It is a light oil which is very moisturising and softening on the skin and the hair. It also helps to relieve inflammation and can be useful for dry, brittle hair and hair that has become lifeless due to chemical and physical stress.

MUSTARD OIL – this oil is often found in Indian grocery stores and is one of the most popular oils used in North-West India. The smell is strong and pungent; its effects are very warming by increasing body heat. It is a popular oil amongst wrestlers and bodybuilders in India. Mustard oil is well known for its ability to break down congestion and swellings from tense muscles and relieve pain. For dryness of the scalp, using mustard oil with a small amount of turmeric powder can prove very effective.

> **CAUTION:** this oil may irritate the skin due to its stimulating nature.

OLIVE OIL – this oil is very popular in the western world. It is of viscous consistency with a strong smell and is therefore often mixed with another lighter oil such as almond. The virgin or extra virgin variety of this oil contains high levels of unsaturated fatty acids and can therefore be useful in helping to moisturise dry skin and hair. It has stimulating properties which help to increase heat in the body and can therefore be used to reduce swellings and alleviate muscular tightness and pain.

SESAME OIL – this is one of the most popular oils used in the western part of India. It is used as a base oils for all oils used in head massage and is very popular in Ayurveda. Sesame seed are high in minerals such as iron, calcium and phosphorus which help to strengthen, nourish and protect the hair. It is an excellent oil for dry skin and hair.

It can also help to improve skin texture, reduce swellings and alleviate muscular pain.

> **NOTE** the oils used in Indian Head Massage are seasonal, with Mustard and Olive being a popular choice in the winter due to their warming effects and Sesame and Coconut being more popular in the summer months.

In addition to the oils mentioned above there are other oils which are traditionally used in India for the treatment of hair. These oils are blended with eastern herbs and spices not readily available in the West. They may be imported and sold in traditional Indian supermarkets and health stores.

AMLA OIL: in combination with henna this is an excellent hair tonic. It promotes the growth of healthy and lustrous hair and has a cooling and nourishing effect.

BRAHMI OIL: this is a unique combination of carefully selected exotic herbs blended with pure coconut oil. Brahmi oil helps the growth of long, lustrous hair and provides relief from dandruff and joint pain.

BHRINGRAJ OIL: this is a popular oil for daily head and scalp massage in India. As well as helping to promote hair growth, it is said to nourish brain cells, help encourage better sleep and relieve stress and tension.

NEEM OIL: this oil is native to India and has antiseptic, astringent and antibacterial properties.

PUMPKIN SEED OIL: this oil is extremely nourishing for dry and stressed hair, as pumpkin seeds are rich in vitamins A, E, C and K, unsaturated fatty acids and proteins.

SHIKAKAI OIL: this is an excellent hair rejuvenator and has stringent and antiseptic properties. Is said to help with eczema and dry scalp.

THE USE OF ESSENTIAL OILS IN INDIAN HEAD MASSAGE

Traditionally essential oils such as Sandalwood, Jasmine and Rosemary have long been used in India as part of Ayurvedic preparations.

Whilst the properties of essential oils can be extremely beneficial to the hair and the scalp, it is recommended that essential oils are not individually blended by a therapist practising Indian Head Massage unless they are qualified and insured for the practice of selecting and blending essential oils. Many essential oils suppliers have pre-blended preparations for sale which may be used in Indian Head Massage.

However, caution is advised on safe proportions due to the fact that when carrying out Indian Head Massage you are close to the brain and the olfactory response, and therefore the effects of essential oils may be enhanced.

Significant Points on the Head for Oil Application in Indian Head Massage

There are three important points on the head according to the Ayurvedic tradition:

1. **THE FIRST POINT** can be found by measuring eight finger widths above the eyebrows. This is where it is recommended that oil is poured onto the scalp initially and then distributed symmetrically down both sides of the head with the fingers.

2. **THE SECOND POINT** is at the crown of the head on the midline: an important therapeutic point and it is where blood vessels, nerves and lymphatics meet. Oil is traditionally poured onto the crown and then evenly distributed down the sides of the scalp.

3. **THE THIRD POINT** is at the base of the skull and is the point the neck meets the skull. Oil is traditionally poured onto this point, with the person's head inclined forwards and then mixed in either side and towards the ears.

Chakra Balancing and Indian Head Massage

Everything that happens to us on an emotional level has an energetic impact on the subtle body, which in turn has an impact on the physical body. Chakras are non-physical energy centres located about an inch away from the physical body. The energy field of each chakra extends beyond the visible body of matter into the subtle body or aura.

It is important to remember that chakras do not have a physical from and any illustration of the chakras is merely a visual aid to the imagination and not a literal physical reality.

Chakras are a way of describing the flow of subtle energy and are often said to be related to an endocrine gland, which the chakra is thought to influence. With stress, the chakras can lose their ability to synchronise with each other and become unbalanced. If negative energy becomes stored in a chakra, it can accumulate and the function of the chakra becomes impaired. Ultimately this can lead to the energy blocks where the chakra virtually ceases to function and creates an imbalance as other chakras attempt to compensate for the blocked centre, creating additional strain for the energy system.

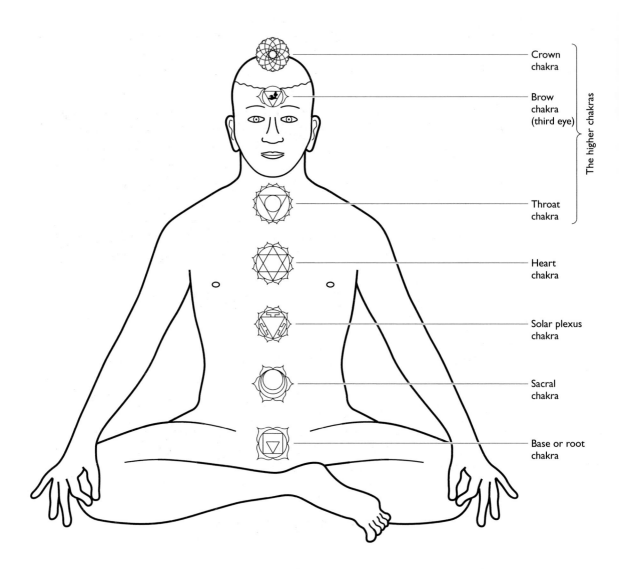

Crown
chakra

Brow
chakra
(third eye)

The higher chakras

Throat
chakra

Heart
chakra

Solar plexus
chakra

Sacral
chakra

Base or root
chakra

The effects of an accumulation of negative energy in the chakras can manifest itself as an emotional or physical condition. Often we are only aware of a change in the physical body as our attention is drawn to it in the form of pain or disease; this may not always be linked to being a symptom of a cause within the subtle body.

Chakras are the focal points for the energies of the subtle bodies and are the key to restoring balancing. By placing hands along the axis of the chakras, energy can be aligned and harmony restored. By working with the subtle energy of the chakras energy may be increased, decreased or balanced as needed by the body at the time of the treatment.

> **KEY NOTE** An important part of Indian Head Massage treatment is the eastern tradition of balancing of the Higher Chakras (the Throat Chakra, the Brow Chakra or Third Eye and the Crown Chakra)
> With stress and tension the chakras lose their ability to synchronise with one another and become unbalanced.
> By placing the hands along the axis of the higher chakras energy can be realigned and a sense of balance and harmony can be restored.

THE THROAT CHAKRA

LOCATION: at the base of the neck
RELEVANCE: this chakra is concerned with communication and expression; it also deals with the issue of truth and true expression of the soul. At a physical level, it is linked to the thyroid and parathyroid glands. Its energies also affect the pharyngeal nerve plexus, the organs of the throat, the neck, nose, mouth, teeth and ears.
IMBALANCE: if this chakra is out of balance it may result in the inability to express our emotions; as a result of unexpressed feeling bottling up, it can lead to frustration and tension. A person with an imbalance in this chakra may feel unable to relax.
COLOUR ASSOCIATION: blue

THE BROW CHAKRA

LOCATION: in the middle of the forehead over the third eye area
RELEVANCE: commonly known as the 'third eye', the brow chakra is the storehouse of memories and imagination and is associated with intellect, understanding and intuition. At a physical level, it is linked to the hypothalamus and pituitary gland. Its energies also affect the nerves of the head, brain, eyes and face.
IMBALANCE: if this chakra is not functioning correctly it can lead to headaches and nightmares. A person with an imbalance in this chakra may be oversensitive to others feelings, be afraid of success, be non-assertive and undisciplined.
COLOUR ASSOCIATION: indigo

THE CROWN CHAKRA

LOCATION: on top of the head

RELEVANCE: this chakra is the centre of our spirituality and is concerned with thinking and decision making. At a physical level it is linked to the pineal gland. Its energies also affect the brain and the rest of the body.

IMBALANCE: an imbalance in this chakra may be reflected in those who are unwilling or afraid to open up to their own spiritual potential. An imbalance may also show as being unable to make decisions.

COLOUR ASSOCIATION: violet

PREPARATION FOR AN INDIAN HEAD MASSAGE TREATMENT

Client Preparation

- Check client is suitable for treatment by carrying out a consultation
- Formulate the client's individual treatment plan
- Seat client comfortably in a chair, ensuring that their legs are uncrossed and feet are placed on the ground
- Drape a towel over the back of the chair and have a clean towel ready for placing over the shoulders for the scalp massage
- Ask the client to remove any obtrusive jewellery such as necklaces, earrings, noserings and to remove glasses
- Ask the client to brush their hair to remove any residue of hairspray and mousse, and to remove face make-up
- If the client's hair is long it should be tied up with a suitable clip

Therapist Preparation

- Present a smart and professional appearance
- Tie hair back off the face
- Remove all obtrusive jewellery and wrist watch
- Ensure chair height is at a suitable height for you and your client
- Prepare oil for the scalp massage, if required (approximately 2-5ml depending on the length of the hair and the condition of the scalp) The oil application is often more preferable when applied to the scalp warm. If this is desired, place the oil container in a bowl of warm water before treatment

Hygiene Precautions

- Cleanse hands before and after treatment
- Check client for any infectious conditions
- Avoid carrying out treatment if you have any infection which may be transmitted
- Cover any open cuts or abrasions with a waterproof plaster
- Pouring oil into a separate container for individual client use and dispose of residual oil

Correct Body Mechanics

Body Mechanics involves the correct use of posture in order to apply Indian Head Massage techniques with the maximum efficiency and with the minimal trauma to the therapist. Therapists often find it more difficult initially adjusting from massaging a client on a couch to massaging a client whilst seated in a chair. It is therefore essential that correct adjustments are made to body mechanics in order to increase the effectiveness of the massage, help prevent repetitive strain injuries, decrease fatigue and increase comfort for the therapist.

Guidelines for correct body mechanics includes:

- Checking chair height – a chair at the correct height will enable a therapist to use body weight effectively to develop pressure.
- Wearing low-heeled shoes with good support
- Keeping the back straight by tilting the pelvis forwards
- Using body weight effectively, by lunging in order to create pressure needed
- Keeping the shoulders and upper back relaxed (avoiding raising shoulders to ears)
- Keeping feet firmly placed on the ground
- Bending knees slightly and keeping knees soft, taking care to avoid locking them straight
- Keeping wrists as straight as possible
- Avoiding joint hyperextension
- Keeping the body in correct alignment by holding head erect over neck and shoulders.
- Keeping head forward posture to a minimum and avoiding spending too much time looking down
- Taking breaks in between clients to stretch the neck, shake out the arms and relax
- Varying the massage techniques used and varying hand and foot placements
- Having regular treatments in order to keep body working at an optimum level

Indian Head Massage Techniques

An Indian Head Massage treatment typically consists of massage to the upper back and shoulders, upper arms, neck, scalp and face. Treatment is traditionally applied through the clothes with the use of oil being optional on the scalp. Illustrated below is an example of a step by step routine of an Indian Head Massage treatment. Due to the fact it has been taught through families for generations and has been westernised, it should be noted that techniques may vary in their content and application.

THE SHOULDERS

The shoulders are the place where most people hold a considerable amount of tension. When the body in a state of tension the shoulders are lifted towards the ears and often remain this way causing the muscles to go into spasm. This restricts the blood flow to the head, neck and shoulders and causes the neck and shoulders to become stiff and inflexible. Sitting with hunched shoulders can reduce chest capacity and thus impair breathing.

> **KEY NOTE** Indian Head Massage can help to counterbalance the effects of stress, as by relaxing the shoulders they will drop and allow the energy to flow more freely to the area, encouraging deeper and easier breathing and improved joint flexibility.

UPPER BACK AND SHOULDER MASSAGE

1) STARTING POSITION WITH HANDS OVER THE TOP OF THE CLIENT'S SHOULDERS

THERAPIST'S STANCE
Standing behind the client in a relaxed posture

TECHNIQUE
Commence by holding your hands lightly on your client's shoulders and ask the client to take 3 deep breaths, with the emphasis of breathing in and out slowly and deeply.

> **KEY NOTE** This helps the client and therapist relax and prepare themselves for treatment.

2) HOLDING POSITION OVER THE TOP OF THE HEAD

THERAPIST'S STANCE

Standing behind the client in a relaxed posture

TECHNIQUE

Hold your hands lightly on top of the head for about a minute, waiting for a feeling of relaxation and calm.

> **KEY NOTE** This helps to create a feeling of stillness and calm before commencing the massage.

3) SMOOTHING ACROSS THE SHOULDERS AND THE UPPER BACK

THERAPIST'S STANCE

Standing behind the client in a walk standing position. Therapists uses walk standing posture to lunge forward and increase the pressure and effectiveness of the techniques.

TECHNIQUE

Use the palmar surface of the hand to mould to one side of the client's back, with the other hand supporting lightly over the top of the opposite shoulder. Use the whole hand to stroke up either side of the spine across the top of the shoulder and around the lateral border of the scapula to return to the starting position with a superficial stroke.

Repeat 3 times one side and then repeat the other side, gradually increasing in pressure with each stroke.

> **KEY NOTE** This technique is the first communication across the shoulders and enables the therapists to establish contact and feel for any areas of tension.

4) SWEEPING ACROSS THE SHOULDERS WITH THE THUMBS

THERAPIST'S STANCE
Standing behind the client in a walk standing position

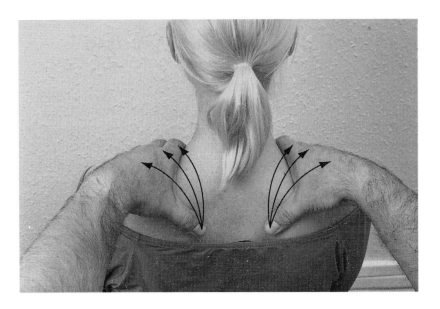

TECHNIQUE
With fingers resting on the client's shoulders, reach down with your thumbs and place them as far as they can go either side of the spine, across the lower border of the trapezius muscle.

Now draw the thumbs up and across the trapezius muscle fanning out towards the little finger. Repeat 3 times, gradually increasing in pressure.

Now draw the thumbs out towards the middle finger and repeat × 3

Then draw the thumbs out towards the index finger and repeat × 3

> **KEY NOTE** This is a deeper technique that helps to unlock tension and free fibrous adhesions from the trapezius muscle.

5) RUBBING WITH THE HEEL OF THE HAND AROUND THE SCAPULAE

THERAPIST'S STANCE
Standing to the side so that you are facing the clients shoulder from the side

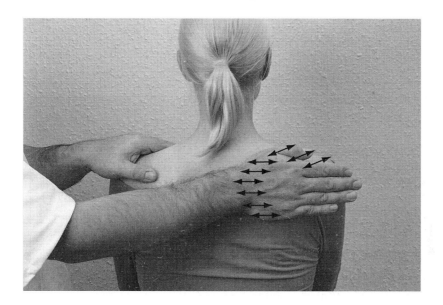

TECHNIQUE
With the heel of your hand rub lightly and briskly (in a side to side motion) across the top of the scapula, in between the scapula and below the scapula in the characteristic 'C' shape . Repeat × 3 each side.

> **KEY NOTE** This technique creates a considerable amount of heat in the tissues and helps to break down fibrous adhesions and restrictions around the scapulae.

6) FRICTIONS AROUND THE SCAPULAE WITH THE FINGERS

THERAPIST'S STANCE
Standing to the side so that you are facing the client's shoulder from the side

TECHNIQUE
Using the fingers joined together (fingertips facing away from the spine) rub vigorously backwards and forwards across the top of the scapula, in between and below the scapulae in the characteristic 'C' shape.

> **KEY NOTE** This technique is similar to the previous technique, in helping to free restrictions and tension from around the scapulae.

7) SMOOTHING EFFLEURAGE

(repeated as in 3)

8) KNUCKLES EITHER SIDE OF THE SPINE

THERAPIST'S STANCE
Standing behind the client in a walk standing position

TECHNIQUE
Using (middle) knuckles of forefinger and middle finger press in slowly and deeply, either side of spine, work from either side of the start of the thoracic vertebrae down to the mid spine. Repeat × 2.

This technique is more effective if the pressure is combined with the client's out breath.

> **KEY NOTE** This technique stimulates the nerve endings either side of the spine, releasing blockages in the nerves and easing tension.

9) THUMB PUSHES OVER THE SHOULDERS

THERAPIST'S STANCE
Standing behind the client in a walk standing position

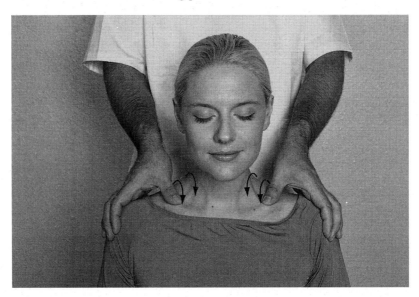

TECHNIQUE
Place the palms of the hands at the corners of the shoulders with thumbs resting above shoulder blades. Starting furthest away from the neck, push the thumbs with medium pressure up and over the shoulder muscles. Repeat × 3

Then repeat at the middle of the shoulders × 3 and at the junction of the neck and shoulders × 3

> **KEY NOTE** This technique loosens tension in the muscles across the top of the shoulders, by squeezing the toxins from the muscle and mobilising the tissues.

10) FINGER PULLS ACROSS THE TOP OF THE SHOULDERS

THERAPIST'S STANCE
Standing behind the client in a walk standing position

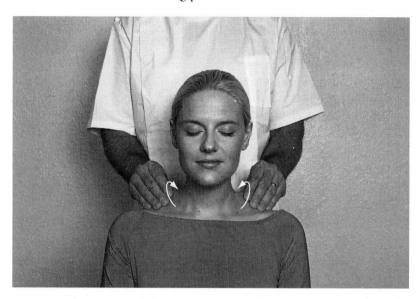

TECHNIQUE
Placing your hands over the top of the shoulders, with the thumbs anchored across the back and the fingers in front of the shoulders.

Pull back with the fingers whilst lifting and squeezing the muscles, drawing the fingers back towards the thumbs.

Repeat several times.

> **KEY NOTE** This technique helps to squeeze the toxins from the muscles fibres and encourage fresh oxygen and nutrients into the muscles. It also helps to soften and loosen the muscles, thereby easing tension.

11) SQUEEZING AND RELEASE ACROSS THE TOP OF THE SHOULDERS

THERAPIST'S STANCE
Standing behind the client in a walk standing position

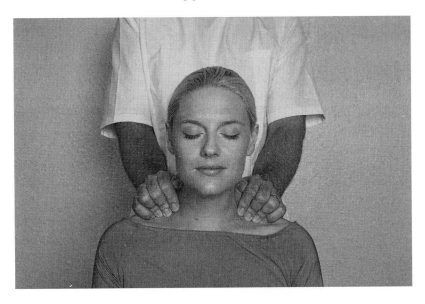

TECHNIQUE
Place palms of hands on the corner of the shoulder with the heel of the hand behind the shoulder muscles and fingers in front. Lift up and squeeze the muscles, clasping them tightly in the palm of the hands by pushing the thumbs towards the fingers, gathering as much muscle tissue as possible. Squeeze using medium pressure and hold for a few seconds. Move further in towards the neck and repeat, gradually increasing the pressure.

> **KEY NOTE** This technique helps to squeeze and release toxins from the muscles, as well as softening and loosening tight muscle fibres.

12) HEEL PUSHES ACROSS THE TOP OF THE SHOULDERS

THERAPIST'S STANCE
Standing behind the client in a walk standing position

TECHNIQUE
Placing hands on top of the shoulders, pick up the tissue as in Movement 11 and then roll the hands forwards across to the front of the shoulders.

> **KEY NOTE** This technique helps to mobilise and loosen the muscles across the top of the shoulders, encouraging the client to release tension.

13) SMOOTHING WITH THE FOREARMS

THERAPIST'S STANCE

Standing behind the client in a walk standing position

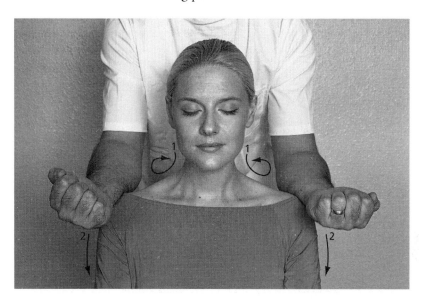

TECHNIQUE

Using the inside of the forearms apply pressure both sides across the top of the shoulders and then glide down across the top of the shoulders and down the upper arms.

i) Starting with fists palm-up at the top of the neck, as arms glide across the shoulders fists should make a half-turn to face palm-down.

ii) Return to palm-up position as fists glide down the forearms.

> **KEY NOTE** This technique stretches and releases the muscles across the top of the shoulders and helps to encourage the drainage of toxins from the tissues. It also encourages the shoulders to release tension.

14) CHOPPING ACROSS THE SHOULDERS AND UPPER BACK

THERAPIST'S STANCE

Therapists position is behind the client kneeling down or standing up with the knees bent, depending on preference and client height.

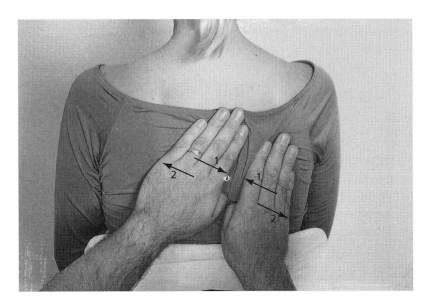

TECHNIQUE

Place the palms of both hands across the shoulders with fingers together and fingertips pointing upwards, perform light brisk chopping movements by quickly moving the index fingers of both hands together and thus picking the tissues up and squeezing them between the index fingers of both hands before releasing them. Work across the whole of the upper back and shoulders.

> **KEY NOTE** This technique helps to loosen the muscles across the upper back and shoulders and stimulates the blood circulation and nerve endings, bringing about a refreshing feeling.

15) HACKING ACROSS THE SHOULDERS AND UPPER BACK

THERAPIST'S STANCE

Standing behind the client in a walk standing position

TECHNIQUE

Using the tips of both fingers, hack up either side of the spine and across the top of the shoulders.

> **KEY NOTE** This technique stimulates the nerve endings and blood circulation, giving a refreshing and revitalising feeling.

16) SQUEEZING ACROSS THE TOP OF THE SHOULDERS

(repeated as in 11)

17) SMOOTHING

(repeated as in 3)

18) HOLDING POSITION OVER THE TOP OF THE SHOULDERS

(repeated as in 1)

Upper Arms

The upper arms are important for upper body movement and when the shoulders are tense they tighten and restrict movement.

When in a state of tension, the upper arms tend to hug the chest either at the sides or in front, whilst the elbows bend up.

> **KEY NOTE** Indian Head Massage can help to reduce tension and tightness in the upper arm muscles to help improve flexibility of the arms and shoulders.

1) SQUEEZING TO THE UPPER ARMS

THERAPIST'S STANCE

Therapist stands to the side of the client, standing behind the upper arms

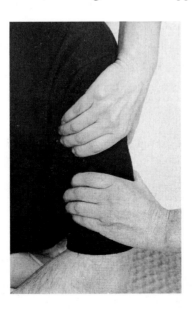

TECHNIQUE

Standing to one side, place the palms of both hands around the upper arm (thumbs resting on triceps and fingertips resting on biceps) and starting at the top of the upper arms, gently squeeze and release, working down the upper arm towards the elbow. Stroke lightly back up to the shoulder and then repeat × 3

> **KEY NOTE** This technique helps loosen tension in the upper arms.

2) SQUASHING TECHNIQUE TO THE UPPER ARMS

THERAPIST'S STANCE

Therapist stands to the side of the client, standing behind the upper arms

TECHNIQUE

With fingers facing towards the floor, place one palm on the anterior surface of the upper arm and one on the posterior surface. Start from the top of the upper arms perform a 'squashing' technique' by gently compressing both palms to squeeze the tissues of the upper arms.

> **KEY NOTE** This technique helps to encourage lymphatic drainage by squeezing toxins from the tissues of the upper arms.

3) HEEL ROLL EMBRACING THE UPPER ARMS

THERAPIST'S STANCE

Standing behind the client in a walk standing position

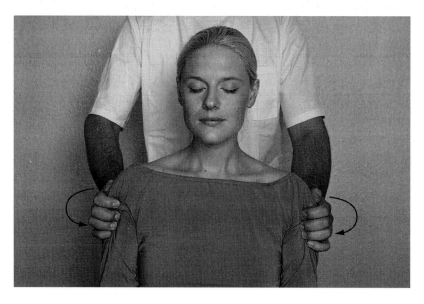

TECHNIQUE

Place your hands on top of the deltoid muscles, fingers in front, heels behind. Roll the heels over the muscles to arrive at your fingertips. Repeat at the middle of upper arm and just above elbow

> ***KEY NOTE*** This technique helps relax and loosen the muscles of the upper arms and top of the shoulder (Biceps, Triceps and Deltoid muscles)

4) SQUEEZING AND KNEADING DOWN THE UPPER ARMS

THERAPIST'S STANCE

Standing behind the client in a walk standing position

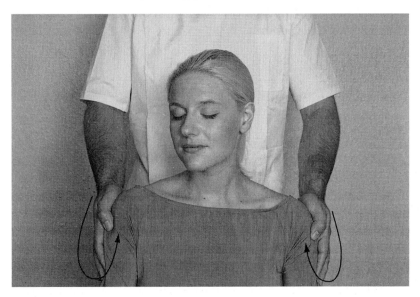

TECHNIQUE

Cup the hands around the cap of the shoulder, thumbs pointing forwards and fingertips behind. Draw your hands from under the back of the client's upper arm and squeeze up and round towards the front of the upper arms. Repeat this movement down to the elbows and then sweep back up to the deltoids and repeat.

> ***KEY NOTE*** This technique mobilises the muscles of the upper arm and helps release tension.

5) GENTLE MOBILISATION TO THE SHOULDER

THERAPIST'S STANCE
Therapist stands to one side of the client, facing the shoulder and upper arm

TECHNIQUE
Stand at client's side, place one hand on the top of the client's shoulder and one hand under the elbow, supporting the clients hand in the crook of your elbow. Gently mobilise the shoulder in a clockwise and anticlockwise direction, trying to take the shoulder its full range of movement.

> ***KEY NOTE*** This technique encourages joint mobility and helps release tension and restrictions in the shoulder joint.

6) SHOULDER LIFT

THERAPIST'S STANCE
Therapist stands behind the client and bends knees

TECHNIQUE
With the client's hands on their lap, place your hands under their elbows and ask the client to take in a long deep breath. As they breathe in pull the shoulder up and outwards and on the client's out breath release the shoulders back down. Repeat this once more.

> ***KEY NOTE*** This technique symbolises letting tension go and helps the clients to drop their shoulders and release the tension.

7) SMOOTHING DOWN THE UPPER ARMS USING THE FOREARMS

THERAPIST'S STANCE
Standing behind the client in a walk standing position

TECHNIQUE
Using the inside of the forearms apply pressure on both sides across the top of the shoulders and then glide down across the top of the shoulders and down the upper arms. Repeat × 3

THE NECK

When the body is balanced, the neck is designed to allow the head to move in a variety of directions. When the body is out of balance and under stress, the head tends to come forwards and the chin juts out. This then throws the body out of alignment as the neck muscles tense and take the weight of the head. The neck muscles are then in a permanent state of contraction and can cause the neck to become stiff and tight. The tension then reduces mobility of the neck and shoulders.

> **KEY NOTE** Working on the neck with Indian Head Massage helps to open up the energy flow from the spine to the whole head and can help to reduce tension, improve posture by re-aligning the muscles, thereby increasing mobility and allowing the head to move more freely.

NECK MASSAGE

1) ROCKING THE HEAD BACKWARDS AND FORWARDS

THERAPIST'S STANCE
Therapist stands to the side of the client

TECHNIQUE
Place one hand on the forehead and one hand at the back of the neck.

Gently rock the head forwards and backwards, taking care to avoid hyperextending the neck. If the neck appears tight, ask the client to breathe deeply 3 times to relax, after which the head should move more freely and with less resistance.

> **KEY NOTE** This technique helps the therapist to assess how much tension there is in the neck and can help the client to relax the neck muscles.

2) KNEADING AND SQUEEZING THE MUSCLES AT THE BACK OF THE NECK

THERAPIST'S STANCE

Therapist stands to the side of the client

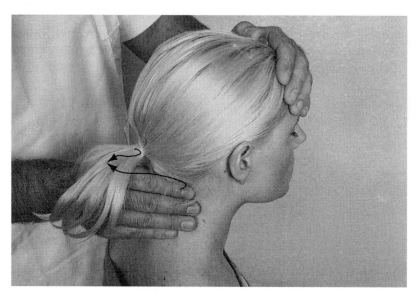

TECHNIQUE

With one hand on the forehead, tilt the neck back slightly and with the other hand spread your thumbs and fingers either side of the base of the neck (forming a V shape). Using firm contact with the skin, slide your hand in to squeeze and lift the muscles of the back of the neck and then release by pulling the hand backwards. Start from the bottom of the neck and gradually work upwards until you reach the base of the skull.

> **KEY NOTE** This technique helps release tension that builds up in the back of the neck and the skull.

3) FINGER FRICTIONS TO THE TOP OF THE SHOULDERS AND UP THE SIDE OF THE NECK

THERAPIST'S STANCE
Therapist stands behind the client to one side

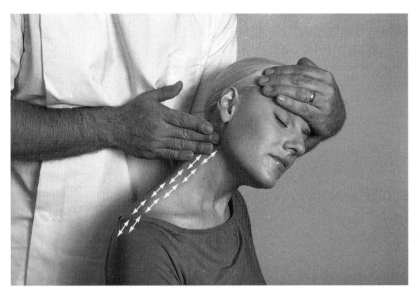

TECHNIQUE
Tilt the client's head gently to one side, supporting the client's head by using the forearm to cup around their head, so that it rests comfortably into the forearm.

Perform frictions using the tips of the fingers in a side to side motion. Start by working across the top of the shoulders and then up the side of the neck to behind the ears.

Repeat 3 times.

Repeat techniques to the other side of the neck

> **KEY NOTE** This technique helps increase the blood and lymph supply to the neck. It also builds up heat in the muscles from the frictions and helps to relieve tightness in the muscles at the side of the neck.

4) THUMB PUSHES TO THE SIDE OF THE NECK

THERAPIST'S STANCE
Therapist stands behind the client to one side

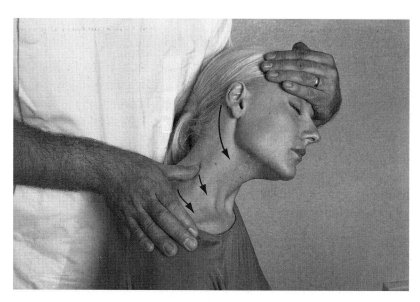

TECHNIQUE
Retaining the same support for the client's head as in movement 3, use the thumb to push deeply into the muscles of the neck by pushing forwards horizontally across from the back of the neck to the side of the neck just below the ears.

Repeat techniques to the other side of the neck

> **NOTE** Caution is necessary during this technique, in order to avoid applying pressure to the carotid arteries at the side of the neck and to respiratory structures such as the trachea on the front of the neck.

> **KEY NOTE** This technique helps to break down fibrous adhesions that restrict movements of the head and neck.

5) SQUEEZING AND RELEASING AT THE SIDE OF THE NECK

THERAPIST'S STANCE

Therapist stands behind the client to one side

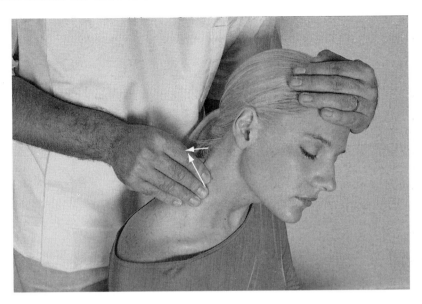

TECHNIQUE

Still retaining the same support for the head as in movement 4, form a V shape between the thumb and the forefinger (thumb is anchored at the back). Squeeze and release the muscles at the side of the neck by lifting the tissue and pulling the forefinger back towards the thumb. Start from the bottom of the side of the neck and work upwards to up behind the ears.

Repeat to the other side of the neck

> **KEY NOTE** This technique helps to squeeze the toxins from the muscles and encourages lymph drainage to the neck.

6) FRICTIONS TO THE BASE OF THE SKULL

THERAPIST'S STANCE

Therapist stands to one side of the client

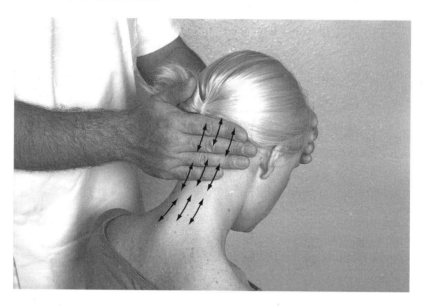

TECHNIQUE

Support the client's forehead with one hand, and use your other hand to perform frictions (with fingers extended) up and down the back of the neck from the base of the neck to the base of the skull.

> **KEY NOTE** This technique helps encourage heat to release tight congested muscles at the back of the neck and the base of the skull, where tension builds up.

7) FRICTIONS WITH THE HEEL OF THE HAND TO THE BASE OF THE SKULL

THERAPIST'S STANCE

Therapist stands to one side of the client

TECHNIQUE

Retaining the supporting hand on the forehead, use the heel of the other hand to apply friction at the base of the skull. Mould the heel of the hand to the base of the skull and use a side to side motion to fiction briskly across the base of the skull.

> **KEY NOTE** This technique helps to encourage the release of toxins from tight congested muscles at the base of the skull.

8) SMOOTHING WITH THE WHOLE HAND AT THE BASE OF THE SKULL

THERAPIST'S STANCE
Therapist stands to one side of the client

TECHNIQUE
Still retaining the supporting hand across the forehead, use the other hand to smooth the base of the skull in a circular motion, repeating several times.

> **KEY NOTE** This technique helps to relax and soothes the neck muscles

9) PRESSURE POINTS AT THE BASE OF THE SKULL

THERAPIST'S STANCE
Therapist stands to one side of the client

TECHNIQUE
Keeping the supporting hand across the front of the head. Use the tip of the middle finger to gently press into the pressure point in the centre of the base of the skull for a few seconds, whilst at the same time gently rocking the head backwards and then move the head forwards to release.

Then using the thumb and the middle finger to press on the points approximately one inch either side of the central point and rock the head gently backwards and then move the head forwards to release.

> **KEY NOTE** This technique helps to relieve pressure from congested nerves and muscles relating to the head and neck.

10) GENTLE STRETCHING TO THE SIDE OF THE NECK

THERAPIST'S STANCE
Therapist stands behind the client to one side

TECHNIQUE
Tilt the client's head gently to one side, supporting the client's head by using the forearm to cup around their head so that it rests comfortably into the forearm.

Place other forearm on top of the client's shoulder and gently press down and hold, before sweeping down and over the top of the upper arm. This movement creates a gentle stretch up the side of the neck.

This movement is enhanced as the stretch is performed on the client's out breath. Repeat to other side

> **KEY NOTE** This technique creates a gentle stretch up the side of the neck.

11) SMOOTHING ACROSS THE BACK OF THE NECK USING THE WHOLE HAND

(repeated as in 8)

THE SCALP

The scalp muscles tighten when under stress, restricting the blood flow, leading to headaches, eyestrain and neck and shoulder tension.

> **KEY NOTE** Indian Head Massage helps to counterbalance stress in the head by improving the circulation and the condition of the hair. Regular head massage also helps to relax the muscles and nerve fibres of the scalp, thereby relieving tension and fatigue.

SCALP MASSAGE

1) RUBBING TO THE SIDE OF THE SCALP, AROUND THE EARS

THERAPIST'S STANCE
Therapist stands behind the client

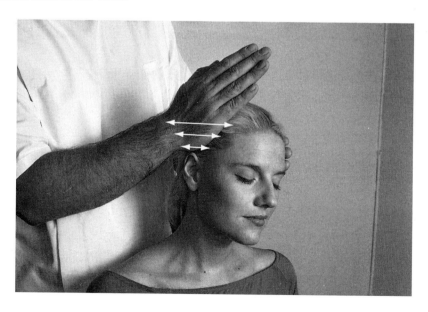

TECHNIQUE

Supporting one side of the head with one hand, use the ball of other hand to carry out light rubbing movements to the part of the scalp above, in front of and behind the ears, with a side-to-side motion, working backwards and forwards.

Repeat to other side

> **KEY NOTE** This technique helps to lightly increase the circulation of blood to the scalp.

2) FRICTIONS TO THE SIDE OF THE SCALP, AROUND THE EARS

THERAPIST'S STANCE

Therapist stands behind the client

TECHNIQUE

Supporting one side of the head with one hand, use 3 fingers extended to perform frictions briskly to the same area as the previous movement (in front of, above and behind the ears). Repeat on the other side of the scalp.

> **KEY NOTE** This technique helps to loosen tension from the temporalis muscle that can cause headaches.

3) RUBBING TO THE WHOLE OF THE SCALP USING THE BALL OF THE HAND

THERAPIST'S STANCE

Therapist stands behind the client

TECHNIQUE

Supporting one side of the head with one hand, use the ball of other hand to carry out rubbing over one side of the head and then the other. Use a broad zigzag motion from side to side working from the front of the scalp towards the back.

> **KEY NOTE** This technique helps to loosen up tight scalp muscles and encourages blood and lymph supply to the scalp.

4) FRICTION TO THE WHOLE OF THE SCALP USING THE WHOLE OF THE HAND

THERAPIST'S STANCE

Therapist stands behind the client

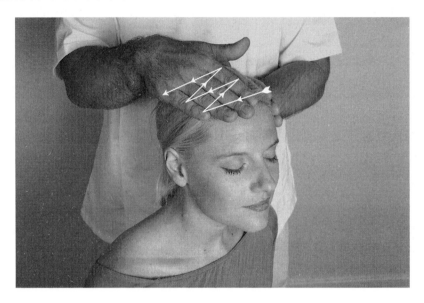

TECHNIQUE

With one side of the head supported, apply firm pressure from the front of the scalp to the back using the whole hand from side to side in a zigzag motion, moving the scalp up and down.

> *Repeat to other side of the skull*

> **KEY NOTE** This technique increases the circulation to the scalp and loosens tight scalp muscles.

5) RUFFLING THROUGH THE HAIR WITH THE FINGERS

THERAPIST'S STANCE

Therapist stands behind the client

TECHNIQUE

Supporting one side of the head with one hand, separate the fingers of the other hand and use the tips of the fingers to perform a light wave-like movement from side to side through the hair from the front of the scalp towards the back.

> **KEY NOTE** This technique has a very soothing and soporific effect on the nerves if performed slowly and is more stimulating and invigorating is performed more vigorously.

6) PLUCKING THROUGH THE HAIR WITH THE FINGERS

THERAPIST'S STANCE
Therapist stands behind the client

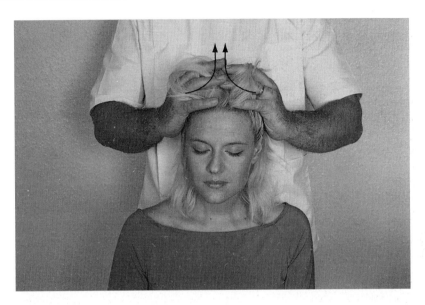

TECHNIQUE
Draw the fingers of both hands through the client's hair, from root to tip in an upwards direction and then release the hair from your fingers, repeating several times. Then gather the hair between your fingers and give the hair a tug to stimulate its growth.

> **KEY NOTE** This technique helps to stimulate the circulation to the scalp and helps bring fresh blood and lymph to the surface.

7) SMOOTHING THROUGH THE HAIR WITH THE FINGERTIPS

THERAPIST'S STANCE
Therapist stands behind the client

TECHNIQUE
Stroke through the hair using the fingertips of alternate hands working repetitively from the front of the scalp towards the back several times.

If your client requires more stimulation to the scalp, use nails of both hands to comb through the hair from front to back.

> **KEY NOTE** This technique has a very calming and soothing effect on the client.

8) TAPPING OVER THE SCALP

THERAPIST'S STANCE
Therapist stands behind the client

TECHNIQUE
Use the fingertips of both hands to perform a light tapping motion over the scalp working from the front of the head towards the back.

> **KEY NOTE** This technique is very stimulating and energising to the scalp.

9) PRESSURE POINTS OVER THE SCALP

THERAPIST'S STANCE
Therapist stands behind the client

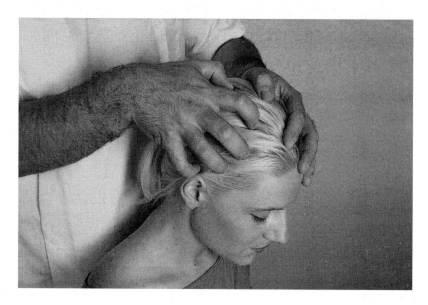

TECHNIQUE
Support the client's head on one side, and with the other hand use the tips of all the fingers and the thumb to perform pressures (with a pumping action) across the scalp, working from hairline towards back of head. Use the fingers and thumb to press in slowly for a couple of seconds and then release.

Work across from one side of the head to the other, changing the supporting hand when you reach the centre of the scalp.

> **KEY NOTE** This technique helps to release blockages from the nerves relating to the head and neck and has a stimulating effect on the head.

10) SQUEEZING THE SCALP MUSCLES

THERAPIST'S STANCE
Therapist stands behind the client

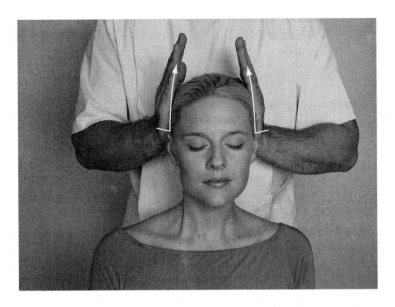

TECHNIQUE
Place your fingers on top of client's head, with the heels of the hands placed behind the ears, elbows apart. Squeeze inward with medium pressure with heels of the hands, lift and release upwards.

Repeat with the heels of hands above the ears and then repeat in front of the ears.

> **KEY NOTE** This technique helps to relieve headaches and eyestrain.

11) CIRCULAR FRICTIONS ACROSS THE TEMPLES USING THE HEEL OF THE HANDS

THERAPIST'S STANCE
Therapist stands behind the client

TECHNIQUE
Support client's head against you and use the heels of both hands to make circular movements against the temples, lifting upwards and backwards.

> **KEY NOTE** This technique is also very effective at helping to relieve tension headaches and eyestrain.

12) SQUEEZE AND RELEASE TECHNIQUE TO THE HEAD

THERAPIST'S STANCE

Therapist stands to the side of the client

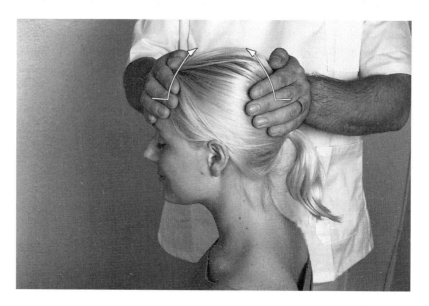

TECHNIQUE

With one hand round front of head and one round the back, squeeze inwards and then release. Repeat 3 times.

> **KEY NOTE** This technique is a very effective technique at helping to release tension headaches.

13) FINISH BY SMOOTHING THROUGH THE HAIR WITH THE FINGERTIPS

(repeated as in 7)

THE FACE

The face is an area of the body that cannot help but show tension. When feeling tense the jaw tends to clamps tight, teeth grind together and the lips tighten.

> **KEY NOTE** Indian Head Massage can help to relax the facial muscles and melt away tension, leaving the client feeling calm and refreshed.

Before commencing the face massage, you may wish to use a dry hand cleanser to cleanse your hands of any oil or sebum that may be left on the hands from the scalp massage.

For the face massage, the client's head needs to be tilted back slightly to rest against therapist's upper thorax.

Ensure that the client's neck is comfortable and offer a neck support or cushion

1) SMOOTHING ACROSS THE FACE

THERAPIST'S STANCE
Therapist stands behind the client

TECHNIQUE
Starting with the fingers across the chin, use the fingers of both hands to smooth up the face with gentle flowing movements, across chin and jaw, across cheeks and across forehead. Repeat 3 times.

> **KEY NOTE** This technique helps to relax and soothe tired facial muscles

2) PRESSURE POINTS ACROSS THE FOREHEAD, AROUND EYE SOCKETS AND AROUND CHEEK BONES

THERAPIST'S STANCE
Therapist stands behind the client

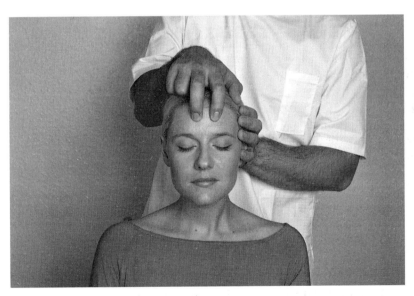

TECHNIQUE
a) Supporting the client's head with one hand, use the pads of the forefinger and middle finger of the other hand to press points in pairs at the midline of the forehead.
PAIR 1: half an inch above the bridge of the nose
PAIR 2: halfway up the forehead
PAIR 3: at the hairline

Then move both fingers outwards approximately half an inch and repeat

b) Then press points on ridge of bone all round the eyes – outwards along the top and inwards along the bottom

c) Now move to points either side of nose and across the curve of the cheekbones and drain sinuses by curving forefingers under cheekbones and holding for a few seconds.

> **KEY NOTE** This technique helps to relieve sinus congestion and encourage lymphatic drainage from the head.

3) CIRCULAR TEMPLE FRICTIONS WITH THE TIPS OF THE FINGERS

THERAPIST'S STANCE
Therapist stands behind the client

TECHNIQUE
With the client's head supported against you, use the fingers to perform circular frictions to the temples, rubbing the area slowly and deeply.

> **KEY NOTE** This technique helps to relieve tension in facial muscles, relieves headaches and eyestrain and helps relax the eyes.

4) MASSAGING THE EARS – SQUEEZING AND TWIDDLING

THERAPIST'S STANCE
Therapist stands behind client

TECHNIQUE
Squeeze the client's ear lobes in between thumb and forefinger, and then release. Then twiddle the ears by rolling the thumb and the forefinger across the ear lobe in a brisk manner.

> **KEY NOTE** This technique stimulates the nerve endings to the whole of the body and creates and energising feeling.

5) SMOOTHING

(as in 1)

6) RELAXING THE FACIAL MUSCLES

THERAPIST'S STANCE
Therapist stands behind the client

TECHNIQUE

Gently place both of your hands so that they cover the lower part of the jaw and cheeks (hands should be barely touching the face and be kept very still, take care not to cover the mouth). From this starting point, gradually move the hands up the face, stopping to place the hands so that the tip of the middle fingers meet at the bridge of the nose. Continue up the face stopping to place the hands so that hands cover the eyes and then continue up the face to finally place hands over the top of the forehead.

> **KEY NOTE** This technique relaxes the facial muscles and the eyes, and creates a feeling of stillness and calm.

7) BALANCING OF THE HIGHER CHAKRAS

THERAPIST'S STANCE
Therapist stands to the side of the client

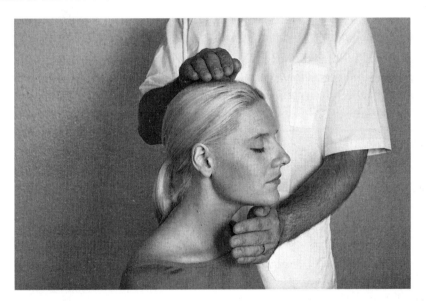

TECHNIQUE
Place one hand lightly over the crown chakra (top of the client's head) and cup the other hand over the throat chakra (without touching throat) and hold hands there for a short while, breathing deeply and slowly to concentrate.

Retaining the hand over the crown chakra, move the other hand up to place lightly over the third eye and hold there for a few moments.

Then place both hands over the crown.

> **KEY NOTE** Chakra balancing helps to re-align the client's energy and is very soothing and calming, helping to bring about a sense of peace and harmony.

8) GENTLE SQUEEZE AND RELEASE TO THE BACK OF THE NECK

THERAPIST'S STANCE
Therapist stands to the side of the client

TECHNIQUE
With one hand over the third eye (brow chakra), spread the thumbs and fingers of the other hand either side of the base of the neck (forming a V shape) and gently squeeze and release the muscles at the back of the neck.

9) RETURN TO THE SHOULDERS TO GENTLY SMOOTH ACROSS THE UPPER BACK AND SMOOTH ACROSS THE UPPER BACK

THERAPIST'S STANCE
Therapist stands behind the client in a walk standing position

TECHNIQUE
Using the palmar surface of the hand, gently stroke up either side of the spine (x 3 each side) and then gently squeeze the top of the shoulders.

> **KEY NOTE** This helps to get the client grounded and bring them back from a deep state of relaxation.

10) SLOWLY LEAVE THE CLIENT'S AURA

After squeezing the top of the shoulders take a step back from the client's aura and gently shake your hands.

Wash your hands

After Care advice

Clients will often feel deeply relaxed following treatment. It is therefore important that clients have a suitable rest period and are offered a glass of water before rising. If oils have been used on the scalp, then clients should be encouraged to leave the oil on for a few hours after treatment before shampooing. When washing their hair after oil application, clients should be advised not to wet their hair first but to apply shampoo to the scalp before the water in order to help to emulsify the oil.

As part of a client's home care programme, therapists may wish to teach clients simple self-massage techniques for the scalp with oils, particularly if the client requires an improvement to their hair condition.

In order to aid the healing process and to get the maximum benefit from their treatments, clients should be advised to:

- increase intake of water following treatment to assist the body's detoxification process
- have a suitable rest period after the treatment
- avoid eating a heavy meal after the treatment; try to keep the diet light whilst the body is using its energy for healing
- avoid smoking
- cut down on consumption of tea, coffee and alcohol
- use oils and simple head massage techniques at home for long term hair care

Reactions to Indian Head Massage

A client's reaction to Indian Head Massage may vary according to their physical and emotional condition. If the body has been under a considerable amount of stress, it is not usual for there to be some kind of reaction as the body adjusts itself back to balance.

Discussed below are some of the reactions that may occur following an Indian Head Massage treatment:

- feeling of tiredness (this is often replaced by a feeling of revitalisation) due to the release of toxins
- relief from stress and muscular tension
- aching and soreness in the muscles due to the release of toxins and the nerve fibres responding to the massage
- an increased feeling of awareness; clients often experience a feeling of calm, peace and tranquillity due to the re-balancing of the chakras
- heightened emotional state
- feeling of alertness and be clearer in mental thought

Adaptations to an Indian Head Massage Treatment

Indian Head Massage, like any other massage techniques, should always be adapted and varied to suit the differences in the physical characteristics of the client, such as body size, muscle tone and age. Therapists are likely to encounter many different clients that may require a degree of adaptation due to their physical and health related situations.

> **KEY NOTE** The best approach to massage is to see every client's situation as a different challenge and view their individual needs as part of the treatment plan. When adapting a massage it is not the massage movements themselves that change; the difference is in the way in which the therapist modifies or adjust the pressure, speed, duration and frequency of the massage.

A pregnant client

It is advisable to avoid carrying out Indian Head massage in the first trimester until the pregnancy is established. The first trimester can be an unsettling time and some clients may experience nausea and sickness.

Once past the first trimester, and provided the pregnancy has no complications, Indian Head Massage can often be a popular choice due to the fact that pregnant clients can sit comfortably in a chair for treatment, and no special positioning is required.

Care should be taken when massaging a pregnant client due to the fact that some clients may experience a feeling of dizziness; care should also be taken, and if necessary, GP referral sought, for those clients who experience high blood pressure during their pregnancy.

A disabled client

The first consideration for the therapist is to establish the nature of the disability, and if necessary research the condition beforehand to be prepared. It is important for a therapist to tactfully enquire about the limitations of the condition and not to assume anything; just because a client is disabled it is does not mean they are paralysed.

If a client is in a wheelchair, then due to the portability of Indian Head Massage they may be treated quite easily whilst sat in the wheelchair.

If the client is in a wheelchair it is advisable for the therapist to sit or kneel when carrying out the consultation in order that they may talk to the client at eye level.

It is essential to take care with disabled clients to not appear patronising, as many disabled clients may be very fit and able and should not be discriminated against because of their disability.

An elderly client

There are several considerations to be borne in mind with an elderly client.
- Take care to ensure the client is warm enough throughout the treatment
- Many elderly people experience a sudden drop in blood pressure, so care needs to be taken to help the client up, to avoid falls and losing balance.

- Avoid deep massage due to decreased reaction time, possible insensitivity to pain and thinning of skin and blood vessels
- There may be loss of hearing and vision
- There will be a decrease in muscle tone and bones will not be as strong and flexible, joints may be worn
- Skin may appear pale, wrinkled, become thinner, looser and more frail.
- The circulation may not be as efficient, especially if the client inactive

It is best to make the treatment sessions shorter as the client may tire easily and to take care when applying pressure and avoid extreme joint mobilisation due to loss of bone integrity.

A Large-Framed Client

Clients with a large frame may find Indian Head Massage more comfortable due to positioning and the fact that no undressing is required.

Pressure should be applied carefully to dense areas of adipose tissue in order to avoid tissue damage and client discomfort. It may be tempting for the massage therapist to consider that areas of fatty tissue are insensitive, and apply too firm a pressure. Adipose tissue is in fact highly vascular, making it highly susceptible to bruising and damage. General pointers are to consider pressure and monitor client feedback and use body mechanics correctly.

The therapist may also need to adjust the chair height depending on the size of the client.

A Small-Framed Client

Care needs to be taken with a thin client to avoid deep massage or pressure over bony areas which may cause discomfort. Stimulating techniques such as hacking should be avoided over unprotected areas, and pressure applied carefully monitored in line with client feedback.

It is important for the therapist to avoid assuming that because the client is thin that they require a light massage; pressure applied should be carefully monitored in line with client feedback.

In general terms the male body presents more muscle bulk than the female body and therefore an adaptation of technique is often required. Male clients will generally require a firmer pressure and the therapist should take care to apply the correct body mechanics and posture in order to be able to carry out the techniques effectively and to the client's satisfaction.

Benefits of Regular Indian Head Massage Treatments

In order to maximise the benefits of Indian Head Massage, it is important for clients to receive regular treatment.

Benefits of regular treatment include:

- improvement in hair condition
- reduction in stress levels
- increased energy levels
- a general sense of well being
- improved sleep patterns
- improvement in circulation

Frequency of Treatment

In India head massage is often part of a daily schedule. In the western world, as part of a stress management programme, Indian Head Massage should ideally be carried out once or even twice a week for maximum benefit. It is advisable to offer clients a course of treatments (between 4 and 6 initially) and to recommend the client takes the treatments close together initially.

Frequency of treatment may vary due to a client's resources, namely time and money, and clients should be encouraged to attend for treatments as frequently as their schedule and financial resources will allow.

Self Assessment Questions

1. Describe the effects of the following techniques used in Indian Head Massage:

a) Rubbing or Frictions

b) Tapping

c) Kneading or Squeezing

2. Describe how a client should be prepared for an Indian Head Massage treatment

3. Describe the beneficial properties of the following oils used for Indian Head Massage

a) Coconut

b) Sesame

c) Mustard

4. Describe 3 reactions which may occur following an Indian Head Massage treatment, explaining why in each case.

5. What after care advice should be given to a client following an Indian Head Massage treatment?

6. How often can an Indian Head Massage treatment be given?

CHAPTER 8

Marketing and Promotion of Indian Head Massage

Marketing is the means by which you tell potential clients what you have to offer and how it will benefit them.

In order to be successful in business, it is not enough for therapists to have excellent skills in the therapy they practice, they also need to get to grips with the important skill of marketing. Holistic therapists need to consider the marketing of services such as Indian Head Massage carefully as they are not looking to sell large volumes of consumer goods; it is a specialist market and the marketing must therefore be selective.

By the end of this chapter you will be able to

- Understand the fundamental issues of marketing and promotion
- Design a marketing plan for business success in Indian Head Massage

Marketing in the holistic therapy industry is educational and is about raising awareness of who you are and what you do. It is important for therapists to consider that marketing is about matching service to clients needs and therefore the focus is not so much on selling but about identifying needs. The key to successful marketing is to view every aspect of your marketing through the client's eyes and match their needs and desires to your products and services.

Marketing involves finding out:
- who your potential clients are
- what their needs are

- how much they would be prepared to pay for the service
- where they are and how to reach them
- how often they would visit

RESEARCHING CLIENTS

It is essential to use market research to assess the needs of the market. Knowing and understanding who your potential clients are is crucial to devising a marketing plan and deciding who to target for advertising and promotion.

Market research enables you to identify potential clients, discover what influences them and find out how to reach them. Knowing the market then enables you to refine the message you wish to send to potential clients. There are very few services that will appeal to everyone; there is always a sector of the market that is going to be more inclined to buy. Therefore, you need to find out who this sector is and focus the attention of your marketing on them.

When building client profiles, it is helpful to consider the following factors:
- age
- gender
- income
- interests
- location

GATHERING CLIENT INFORMATION

As clients are at the centre of every business, it is vital to find out about them and what they want. Carrying out marketing surveys using questionnaires are an effective way of gathering information. A great deal of thought needs to be given to the design of a marketing questionnaire in order to give both quantitative and qualitative results.

When designing marketing questionnaires, it is important to keep questions short, simple and to the point in order to get an exact answer. If questions are structured it is simpler and quicker for the respondent to reply. Another important consideration is in the type of questions to ask. Closed questions only require yes/no/don't know response and open questions are such as that the respondent has to answer in their own way.

It is also important to remember when designing questionnaires to avoid pre-judging the participant's response, in other words not assuming that you know what they are going to say. Neither should you leave them with no alternative but to agree with you.

In order to get the best results from your marketing questionnaire bear in mind the following:

- keep it simple, attractive, interesting and relevant
- include a short introduction to the questionnaire in order to stimulate the respondents' enthusiasm and motivation to complete it
- offer an incentive to complete the questionnaire (such as a free prize, or entry into a free prize draw)
- make it known to the respondents that there is a deadline for reply to the questionnaire

You may wish to carry out a pilot survey on a group of individuals (friends, family, colleagues); however, check the individuals concerned are amongst the right category of a potential client, otherwise this may be prove to be a fruitless exercise.

Opposite is an example of a market research questionnaire for Indian Head Massage.

Client surveys are useful tools in market research in that by gaining the client's input they:

- demonstrate your desire to offer the best possible service
- help you to fulfil the client's needs
- direct you towards potential sales triggers
- guide you towards potential strengths and weaknesses

If sending out market research questionnaires, always make the response easy for the client by providing a stamped addressed envelope.

As Indian Head Massage involves a personal and specialised service it tends to appeal to certain segments of the market. By selecting a target market it enables you to modify your advertising and promotional activities to appeal to a specific group.

Consider the type of clientele you want to attract or if you have an existing clientele examine who is already using your services and what they have in common.

When targeting client markets it is wise to have more than one sector, the number being dependent on your preference, expertise and the size of your practice.

In order to make marketing more effective, it is helpful to create a niche market by addressing the needs of a specific group of people. Your name then becomes linked with providing a particular service for a particular target group.

ASSESSING MARKETING NEEDS

Marketing needs will be dependent on the following factors:

- your target market
- the size of your practice
- the amount of money you can afford
- the amount of time you can devote.

Indian Head Massage Questionnaire

Indian Head Massage is a traditional massage treatment originating from India. It involves the application of massage techniques to the upper back and shoulders, upper arms, neck, face and scalp. The treatment is applied through the clothes, with the recipient remaining seated in a chair.

Indian Head Massage has many benefits including helping to relieve muscular tension, relieving headaches reducing stress levels.

This questionnaire is designed to establish current levels of awareness and interest in Indian Head Massage.

1. Have you heard of Indian Head Massage before?   **Yes/No**

2. If Yes, when did you hear about it?

_____

_____

3. Do you experience any of the following on a regular basis?

high stress levels? ☐   muscular tension in the back, neck or shoulders? ☐

headaches? ☐   eyestrain? ☐   anxiety? ☐   depression? ☐

poor concentration levels? ☐

4. What measures do you take (if any) to help with any of the following?

_____

_____

5. Would you be interested in trying a treatment?   **Yes /No**

6. Would you like further information on Indian Head Massage and its benefits?

Yes/No

Thank you for your time and co-operation in completing this form. If you would like further information or would like to book a complimentary introductory treatment, please give your details below.

Name _____

Address _____

Telephone Number   Work: _____ Home: _____

If you are a therapist starting out in business and do not have a large clientele, more time and energy can be devoted to making contacts, giving talks and presentations to help get your name and what you do known. The activities involving client education and awareness will be low cost but time consuming.

If you are an established business you may have the financial budget to concentrate on other marketing methods such as targeted advertising or mailshots to announce a new service such as Indian Head Massage into the business. An important factor to consider in marketing is that it takes time and money to become known in business.

Compiling a Marketing Plan

Once you have established where the market for Indian Head Massage is and how extensive it is, the next stage is to put all the findings together in the form of objectives – this will form a marketing plan. A marketing plan will form the basis of how you intend to promote the service to generate clients. Before compiling a marketing plan, it is essential to carry out a **SWOT** analysis in order to self-assess your Strengths, Weaknesses, Opportunities and Threats in order to be realistic in your plan.

STRENGTHS – these may include
- specialism
- location of the business
- pricing
- the opening hours
- personality
- customer service
- flexibility

> **KEY NOTE** A marketing plan should also include your Unique Selling Position (USP) which is what makes your business and service different.

WEAKNESSES – Possible weaknesses may be
- lack of experience
- opening hours
- location
- range of skills offered

OPPORTUNITIES – This could include:
- expansion into other sectors of the market i.e. the workplace

THREATS – Potential threats may include:
- local competition

Getting the Balance Right in Marketing

Successful marketing usually involves a mix of different methods and the chemistry or 'mix' has to be right for the individual business.

Marketing can be divided into four factors and each of these will influence how you develop your marketing plan. Marketing can be seen as a balancing act and if adjustments are made to one or more of the four factors, then a similar adjustment has to be made on the other factors in order for the approach to be balanced.

PRODUCT/SERVICE – this includes the features and benefits of the product/service being offered, including the quality of service. For marketing to be effective it is important to create a demand.

With products and services, it is also important to consider the image of the business being projected by the service itself, the marketing material and the staff.

PRICE – this is the cost of the service to the client. When setting prices for services it is vital to consider the following:
- charge enough to cover your overheads and enough to meet your expenses and make a profit
- charge what clients are prepared to pay
- be in line with your competitors

PLACE – this is where you are located in relation to your clients. Careful consideration needs to be given to the location and opening hours of the business to ensure the service is available to potential clients.

Location is an important factor in business that affects the distribution of services.

Due to the portable nature of Indian Head Massage therapists should consider the many locations or settings in which the therapy may be practised (i.e. in the workplace, in hairdressing salons and hospitals as well as beauty spas and clinics).

PROMOTION – The objective of promotion is to become known and to create a desire in potential clients to use your services.

The promotion of services such as Indian Head Massage is largely educational in nature and is the means by which potential clients learn who you are, what you do and how your services will benefit them.

In the Holistic Therapy industry it is important for therapists to realise that they are marketing themselves as well as their treatments.

Marketing is the art of promoting yourself and the services you offer in order to attract clients.

There are many marketing strategies that can be used to sell the services you intend to offer, however one of the most important attributes for a holistic therapist is to have self confidence, a positive attitude and belief in themselves and their abilities.

As the holistic therapy business is a personal service it is essential that therapists feel confident enough to sell their services and products to potential clients.

In order to be able to sell a service or product effectively it is important for a therapist to :
- know the services well enough and have enough experience to be able to sell their benefits to potential clients
- be aware of the services of competitors and have identified their strengths and weaknesses
- be able to sell solutions
- identify with the potential clients needs and personalise the sale

Personality Selling

The concept of personality selling is very important in business. Some clients may decide whether to have a treatment based on factual information. In this case benefits of the treatment need to be stressed in a very factual and analytical way.

Other clients may need to have a picture created for them enhanced by imaginative therapeutic words to stimulate their interest.

> **KEY NOTE** Some therapists may feel uncomfortable with the idea of selling and may need to attend sales training in order to enhance this very important skill.

No amount of advertising can make up for the personal touch and with Indian Head Massage it is best to consider the direct and more personal approach first and turn personal skills to your advantage. By creating a positive environment for treatment provision, therapists can sell through one of the most powerful senses – the therapeutic touch. When planning advertising and promotion, it is essential to use a mix of methods in order to reach different target markets and to help evaluate the overall effectiveness of the activities.

The Direct Approach to Marketing and Promotion

Personal Recommendation/Word of mouth

This is the most valuable form of advertising for personal treatments like Indian Head Massage. Once a therapist has established a reputation for excellent customer service and quality skills, a satisfied client will automatically recommend the service to another potential client. It is important for therapists to tell as many people as possible about Indian Head Massage and communicate their enthusiasm. Positive enthusiasm is infectious and even if the person you are speaking does not need the information they may pass it on to someone who does. The power of the spoken word is very effective in the marketing of services.

Talks and Demonstrations

Talks and demonstrations are an effective way of presenting the service to a targeted group and they usually work best when presented together.

Talks should be informative and educational in nature (they should tell potential clients how it will benefit them) and the demonstration will show the target audience the effects and will help to break down barriers or pre-conceptions they may hold about the therapy.

It is useful to identify the needs of target audience prior to the presentation of group as it gives the therapist the advantage of being able to personalise the session.

Talks and demonstrations are better being limited to a maximum of 30-40 minutes, with time left to answer questions and to distribute business cards and literature.

The focus of the talk should be about identifying with and providing solutions to the client's needs.

A useful checklist when preparing for talks is to:
- find out as much as possible about the target group before the talk
- confirm the number of people that will be attending
- check out the venue and its suitability
- plan out the talk with a basic outline format
- have a plentiful supply of literature to hand out
- prepare a list of possible questions you may be asked
- take some relaxation music to help create a relaxing ambience
- aim to involve the audience in the session (encourage questions or use of them to demonstrate on)
- take your appointment book with you!

Exhibitions

Exhibitions are an effective way to communicate with lots of potential clients in one place. It is a useful way of distributing brochures and leaflets and to persuade new clients to watch a demonstration of a new service and sample it. When exhibiting at a show it is important to ensure that it is the right type of show for the image of the business of therapist and to speak to people who have attended the show in order to gain feedback from them.

In order to project the right image at an exhibition it is important to ensure that
- The stand is accessible and situated to your best advantage
- That staff manning the stand look warm and welcoming, and are approachable to talk to
- That the stand looks attractive, neat and tidy
- There is space for people to browse without feeling intimidated

It is also important, if possible to take the names and contact numbers of those who visited the stand in order that you may contact them after the exhibition.

Building a Referral Network

This is one of the most successful and inexpensive ways of creating new business.

Current satisfied clients are one of the most effective means of advertising.

Referrals can be encouraged by:
- offering existing clients incentives to introduce new clients to use your service
- establishing links with other professionals by making yourself and what you do known to them

Public Relations

This is a way for therapists to get their name in the public eye without actually paying for advertising.

There are a variety of ways in which it can be done.
1. Offering a free talk and demonstration to a particular client group in the community is an ideal way of marketing Indian Head Massage and helping to get your name and reputation established.

    Public interest in holistic therapies is increasing all the time and there are many groups that meet regularly who may be keen to hear from you (a list of contact names, addresses and phone numbers may be obtained from your local library).
    See talks and demonstrations (page 000).
2. Sending information or news concerning your business to editors of newspapers or magazines in the form of a news article. Everyday editors and journalists are looking for stories and information to fill their newspapers or magazines.

    An important consideration when sending information to journalists is to only send information that it truly of interest to the community and their readers.
3. Donating your time, money or products to a local worthwhile charity. There are many charitable organisations who rely on donations each year to survive. An event linked to funding or sponsoring a charity would be a newsworthy article, as well as helping to meet the needs of the community.
4. Getting a regular or one-off slot on the Local Radio (see Local Radio page 000).

5. Compiling a press release which may be sent to local and national newspapers and magazines.

When compiling a press release the following guidelines may help to increase your chance of publication:
- think of an original, interesting, thought-provoking or even humorous headline
- avoid trying to sell your service
- it should be newsworthy and of interest to the journalists and their readers
- address the information directly to a named editor or journalist, preferably one you have already established contact with
- ensure that it is laid out clearly (preferably double-line spacing) and is no longer that two pages
- always include a contact name, address and telephone number

> **KEY NOTE** Editorials in the newspapers and magazines are seen to be credible and true as readers place a considerable amount of trust in the objectivity of journalists. It is therefore worth getting to know editors and journalists and being persistent, as the articles they write tend to hold a lot of weight with readers.

Indirect approach to Marketing and Promotion

There are several other methods of advertising or marketing which may be used in order to reach the potential clients you cannot reach in person and these include:
- Newspaper Advertising
- Specialist magazines
- National directories
- Mailshots
- Leaflets and promotional material
- The Internet
- Local Radio
- Cross merchandising promotional literature

Advertising strategies usually involve a mix of different media and should be scheduled over a period of time for maximum effects. Isolated advertisements rarely sustain enough interest.

Advertising is about getting your message across. Important considerations when considering an advertisement are:
- What do you want to say to potential clients?
- Who is your target audience?
- How you will communicate to them what you want to say

It is essential to follow the tried and tested **AIDA** formula when considering your publicity:

A – attracting **ATTENTION** – this can be created by an appropriate heading that attracts attention
I – generating **INTEREST** – this can be created by stating what is on offer
D – creating **DESIRE** – this can be created by stating why what you have to offer is needed and getting potential clients to believe in the benefits
A – motivating **ACTION** – this can be created by offering the reader an incentive (special offer)

Good advertisements are usually targeted to the right audience; accurate and not misleading; catchy, concise and memorable. Effective adverts must have a good headline (select a major benefit for this) to have immediate impact. A good headline will:
- attract reader's attention
- compel the person to read further
- improve response
- express the most important benefits

A good advert should be easy to read and be written to
- touch peoples emotions
- be informative
- promote the service
- raise awareness
- motivate reader to act

When designing adverts, ask yourself what adverts you responded to and why.

KEY NOTE Words that tend to sell in adverts include:
You, New, Results, Health, Free, Complimentary, Benefits, Now, Yes

---

Local papers

There are two types of advertisements in newspapers and these are display advertisements and business classified. Display advertising is more expensive and could appear anywhere in the paper, unless you have paid to have a particular space such as the front of back page, or the television page (which could prove very expensive).

It is always a gamble when relying on display advertising as it may be largely dependent on the following:
- The day of the week the paper is printed
- The time of the year
- The page the advert appears on
- The layout of the advert in relation to the other advertisers

An important point to consider with display advertising is that people buy papers for many reasons other than to read adverts (reading news, announcements and events, crosswords, horoscope). It is therefore important to consider how your advert is going to grab their attention, bearing in mind that newspapers have a short life span and bearing in mind the AIDA principle.

It is also useful to consider that the person reading the news and features may come across your display advert and may not be thinking about a massage until he or she sees your advert, or they may not be ready to have a massage for some while. In fact it may take many exposures to your advert before this person feels you are sufficiently familiar to give you a try. It is important therefore that adverts are repeated regularly in the same way in order to create familiarity. It can also help to have a picture of yourself in the advert as it will be more eye-catching and will help the potential client to feel they know you.

It is important to remember when writing adverts that you are speaking directly to your potential clients and the reader will be initially attracted by your headline message, rather that the name of your business. It is often helpful to give the reader a cause to reply now, such as a deadline on a special offer, as this motivates action.

When you have designed an advert, it is often helpful to ask friends and colleagues to cast an eye over the design and the wording for critical review; often a fresh pair of eyes can help add constructive comments.

Display advertising is usually more effective when it is combined with some editorial. Often papers run special features on Health related matters and it may be more appropriate to consider a display advert within a feature as it draws the reader's attention to a more focused subject. Classified advertising is more cost-effective than display advertising as it is more targeted to the service to be provided. The disadvantage with classified is that there may not always be an appropriate section for holistic therapies and advertising will need to be placed frequently in order to make it effective.

Specialist Magazines

These are usually targeted to a specific audience and the ones related to health are those normally of interest to a holistic therapist. The main drawback with them are that they are not local but national and will depend on the readership and the location of the therapist as to whether the advertising will be effective.

> **KEY NOTE** Check the readership profile before committing to advertising in magazines and check circulation radius and readership numbers.

Promotional Material

When writing and designing promotional material the key to success is to write it as if you know the client personally. Choose words carefully in order that they strike a chord with the client.

Remember that many clients reading promotional material may not know they are looking for your service until they see it.

It is also important to consider when developing marketing material to ensure that it reflects the image you wish to portray and that it appeals to the target market.

Promotional materials such as leaflets, brochures and posters are the means by which clients will decide whether to contact you for an appointment. Promotional materials must be attractive enough to make then read it and wording should be positive, direct and above all personal. Brochures and posters with a question and answer format can help clients to overcome their objections and visual aids can help to attract attention.

It is also important to use positive language and turn a negative statement (such as a client's problem) into a positive one (how your treatment is going to help them). Including testimonials from satisfied clients (with their permission) can also help to build credibility and break down barriers.

Mailshots

Mailshots can be a worthwhile exercise but require a degree of planning and forethought. It is far more effective to target a specific group when designing a mailshot, as the main theme is to address the needs of all the respondents.

You may choose to target self-help groups with a common need of relaxation or may choose to write to the Occupational Health Advisor at local companies offering to give free talks and demonstrations as part of their stress management programme.

The letter should be sent on headed note paper and be brief and concise. The focus should be on the respondents needs, although it is helpful to send background information on yourself and your background along with information on Indian Head Massage.

Mailshots usually have a success or response rate of around 2%, although this may be enhanced to 5% by follow-up phone calls.

> **KEY NOTE** When writing to companies it is worth offering the incentive of corporate membership, as a promotion to motivate more clients to use your service. Each employee may be issued with a corporate membership card which entitles them to a certain percentage of discount.

When sending a mailshot it is important to consider the day it is mailed out as this could have a significant effect on the result. If sending a mail shot to clients homes, aim to send it to arrive on a Friday or Saturday ready for the weekend, when they may have more time to consider what you are offering. If sending mail shots to companies, aim to send the information to arrive on a Tuesday or Wednesday and not on a Friday or Monday.

Getting Corporate Clients

Indian Head Massage is ideally suited to the workplace due its unique selling points

- It is portable in nature
- It is quick
- It provides a solution to client's problems
- It is a personal service
- There is no need for the client to undress
- No special resources are required

If your objective is to secure contracts with corporate clients, firstly consider which companies (both large and small) are within your catchment area and the profile of the staff members.

When approaching corporate clients, it is important to create a corporate image for yourself, even if you are not part of a large organisation. The first point of contact should be by letter directly to the person within the organisation who is responsible for the health and welfare of staff (this may an Occupational Health Advisor, Staff Nurse, Health and Safety Office or Managing Director). The letter should be sent on quality headed note paper; the main theme of the letter should be focused on the workplace benefits of Indian Head Massage and how it can benefit the staff and the organisation (see stress management chapter). When approaching corporate clients it is advisable to avoid 'flowery' therapy language and be specific and accurate in terms of the outcome (the benefits). Offer to come in and give a free talk and demonstration with no obligation. Once the letter has been sent, keep a record of it and follow it up with a phone call approximately seven to ten days after.

Remember that businesses, whether large or small, receive a lot of paperwork to read through the post. Do not assume that the reason you have not heard from them is that they are not interested. They may simply not have had the time to read your letter.

Publications and Directories

Advertising in national publications and directories such as Yellow Pages can be an effective way of advertising, as it is targeted to a specific skill area by virtue of the fact it is classified by therapy type. It is also a long-term form of advertising and can prove to be cost-effective as it is a yearly publication.

Therapists should also consider their geographical location and if they are situated between two counties, it may be advisable to take an advert in more than one directory.

If there are several therapists advertising under the same category then it is important to consider your USP (unique selling point) and stress this in order to give a point of difference from competitors.

Internet

Some therapists are now taking advantage of the internet as a means of advertising their treatments. An attractively designed web page including a treatment menu and a photograph of the therapist can all be factors that may enhance contact from any interested parties. It can also help to give a therapist a more corporate image, which is especially important if it is this sector of the market you are interested in pursuing.

Some feel that the internet is a little impersonal but others who are constantly using it feel it is a very efficient means of communication.

It is certainly worth considering this as a potential source of enquiries and contact, but remember that not everyone will have access to the internet and may prefer the more traditional means of contact.

Radio

Radio is an excellent form of media in raising awareness of treatments such as Indian Head Massage.

Consider contacting your local radio station with a view to having either a regular or one-off spot on the radio to promote Indian Head Massage. It is important when approaching the station to make the proposal interesting and one which will interest their listeners. It is important to respond to local trends or issues (for instance lifestyle or reducing stress) when presenting information on the radio, as it has to be topical and of value to listeners. Assessing growth trends within the industry will help you to assess the opportunities afforded to you.

When preparing to talk on the Radio it is important to find out as much as possible about the programme you will be appearing on, the profile of the listeners and most importantly the style of the Radio Presenter. Some presenters prefer to work to a script and will run through a list of questions before the programme, others prefer to work unscripted and make the presentation more spontaneous.

> **KEY NOTE** Local Radio stations often look for gifts that can be given to listeners in exchange for on-air promotions. Donating your services is an easy and effective way of getting your name out on the airwaves without buying advertising time.

Cross-Merchandising Promotional Literature

Consider other local businesses that cater to clientele similar to yours (i.e. hairdressers, osteopaths, etc) and who may be in a position to influence clients to try Indian Head Massage.

Exchange promotional literature and brochures with them and this will allow each party additional exposure to the type of clients they wish to attract. When approaching other local businesses with a view to cross-merchandising, it is important to establish a friendly, approachable and co-operative working relationship, as this will enhance the success of the promotion on both sides.

Encouraging Client Retention

The first goal of marketing is to encourage potential clients to try out your services; the next goal is to encourage them to come back again. There are two main ways of fostering repeat business:

- creating an understanding of the benefits of the treatments you provide to clients by encouraging them to book regular treatments
- awarding loyalty bonuses and reward schemes (such as ones offered by major supermarket chains)
- staying in touch with your clients and informing them of special offers and any new treatments you may have added to your treatment menu (and how they can benefit them)
- inviting clients to attend talks and events you may be holding

Maximising Marketing Opportunities

Due the widespread appeal of Indian Head Massage it is well suited to clinics, salons and spas, as well as other associated trades such as hairdressers, osteopaths, chiropractors and health clinics. Consider all places where people attend regularly for reasons of health, beauty and relaxation.

A local hairdressers may be interested in adding Indian Head Massage to their treatment menu to give a different marketing angle to their customer service.

Osteopaths and chiropractors may be interested in Indian Head Massage for clients with soft tissue problems of the head, neck and shoulders.

A GP surgery may be interested in helping clients with stress, anxiety and depression or people with musculo-skeletal problems.

If you have a local regional airport nearby, they may be interested in a business proposal to offer treatments to tired business executives in need of stress relief.

A local school may benefit from a regular visit to help teachers and students to manage their stress levels.

If you use your imagination, there are a multitude of different opportunities and reasons for marketing Indian Head Massage.

Selling of Associated Products

As providing treatments are a labour intensive service consider selling complementary products for client's home use. Clients are more likely to buy products such as scalp oils and relaxation tapes at the time of their treatment. It is therefore advisable to have a display of items available for purchase at reception or wherever the client is likely to pay. Clients are also more likely to buy from their therapist, with whom they have a trusting relationship.

Creative Marketing Opportunities

Other creative marketing opportunities could be to offer gift certificates linked to promotions at specific times of the year such as Christmas, Valentines Day, Birthdays, Mothers Day or Fathers Day. Specially packaged courses of treatments often attract interest as they are designed specifically to address the needs of the respondents.

Male Clients

An area that it is often left unexploited is the market of male clients. Marketing treatments such as Indian Head Massage can require a different strategy to selling to female clients.

Men often respond more to factual and benefit related words rather than the more kinaesthetic language women tend to respond to. Think of male dominated markets and how that target may be reached. Local sports clubs and associations may be a good start, men's barbers, health clubs.

An important consideration when marketing to male clients is to consider whether the environment you are practising in is male-friendly (it will be difficult to attract male clients into a salon that looks too pretty). Some men are also conscious of their body image; it may therefore be more prudent to schedule specific times for male clients to attend.

DEFINING MARKETING OBJECTIVES

Once you have put together the right mix of marketing methods, the next stage is to define your marketing objectives. Marketing objectives are closely linked to overall business objectives and will define what you want to achieve from your marketing and how you intend to meet the objectives.

Example of Marketing Objectives for a therapist practising Indian Head Massage:

Objectives

Short Term

1. To introduce Indian Head Massage to existing clientele

Medium Term

2. To expand the existing client base to secure new clients

Long Term

3. To introduce Indian Head Massage into the workplace

Strategy

1. Send a newsletter to all existing clients advising them of the benefits of Indian Head Massage and how it can help them. Include a voucher with a special introductory offer.

2. Contact the editor of a local newspaper to offer an article on Indian Head Massage that is going to be of interest to readers and a free demonstration.

3. Write to 20 local companies with an short but informative introductory letter. Offer a corporate discount. Follow up with a phone call in 7-10 days with a view to securing a meeting to offer a free talk and demonstration.

Monitoring Marketing Methods

It is important to regularly monitor the response to marketing methods, to help you assess which methods are working to help you meet your business objectives.

It is essential to constantly monitor, review and adapt your strategies in order to ensure continued business success. Marketing methods may change with a difference in trend or may simply become out-dated.

A simple and effective way of monitoring the response to your marketing methods is to ask each new client how they heard of you and keep a record of this in order to review it in line with your business objectives. Provided you know how much a particular method cost and how many clients were generated from it, you are then in a position to analyse which methods are cost-effective.

Once you establish a clientele you can then build up information such as how often they attend for treatments, how much they spend and what marketing methods they respond to.

For marketing to have the desired effects it should be
- **SUFFICIENT** – it has to be done regularly, even when you are busy
- **EFFICIENT** – it has to be cost-effective to be worthwhile
- **EFFECTIVE** – it has to work and get results

HOW TO ENCOURAGE REPEAT BUSINESS

Maintaining excellent customer service is the key to encouraging repeat business.

It is important to make it easy for clients to come to you by:
- making client needs a priority
- concentrate all your actions and efforts for the business with the client in mind
- treating every client like a new client and avoiding complacency
- delivering an excellent service
- building an open relationships with clients by encouraging feedback

Keeping Ahead of Business

Many businesses fail to realise their potential because they don't continually market their business. An important factor to consider is that many clients may have to see your advert or marketing material many times before responding.

Many therapists fail to be consistent in marketing methods believing they already have enough clients. Even if the appointment book is full, it is important to keep on marketing to raise client awareness and maintain your professional image, as you never know when you are going to lose current clients due to various circumstances (client personal or financial circumstances, client moving out of the area etc).

How is Indian Head Massage different to ordinary massage?

The first main difference is that the client remains fully clothed throughout the treatment.

The treatment can be given with the client sat in an ordinary chair, as long as it is comfortable.

The client does not have to lean forward either as they will remain in a normal seated position during the treatment.

A traditional treatment will also involve the balancing of the Chakras.

It is extremely popular with all types of clients and is an ideal treatment for pregnant clients or for clients who are disabled, due to the position of the client during treatment.

STRESS IN TO-DAY'S SOCIETY

Stress is now widely regarded as the Public Health enemy Number One.

Indeed, according to Management Today, one report from the California Institute of Technology suggested that roughly 80% of individuals who attend Doctors' surgeries do so because of stress-related diseases.

The ever-rapid increase of Modern Technology enables people to undertake more each day.

Such increase brings in its wake additional **STRESS** and many observers believe that **STRESS** will continue to increase.

Indian Head Massage is predicted to become one of the **fastest growing stress management treatments** of the New Millennium.
It is proving to be an extremely valuable element of stress management programmes due to the benefits it produces and also it's simplicity and ease of application.

Who do I contact for further information

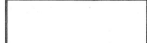

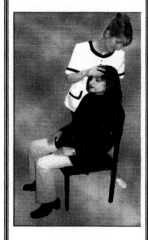

Indian Head Massage

A Brief Guide

Indian Head Massage ...

... is a traditional Indian technique of treating the upper back, neck, shoulders, face and scalp, with the recipient remaining clothed.

The techniques were originally developed by women who used oils, such as sesame, coconut and mustard oil to help keep the hair strong, lustrous and in beautiful condition.

In India, a head massage is traditionally performed as part of the treatment given by barbers and masseurs and is commonly seen being performed on street corners, markets and the beach.

How does it work?

Indian Head Massage works on both a physical and psychological level, the techniques used represent a de – stressing programme for the whole body.

By massaging the head and shoulders, energies will become rebalanced and a general feeling of relaxation will be achieved for the whole body.

Indian Head Massage can improve blood flow to the head and neck, which increases the distribution of nutrients to encourage healing within the whole body.

What does a treatment involve?

Treatment, is carried out to the upper back, across the shoulders, upper arms, neck, scalp and face, with the client remaining fully clothed and seated in an everyday chair.

Because the treatment is non – invasive, it may be undertaken anywhere.

The use of oils on the scalp is optional.

What are the Benefits ?

It can help to:

- relieve eyestrain and headaches

- improve concentration

- relieve physical and mental fatigue

- improve joint mobility

- relieve stress and muscular tension

As well as being a relaxing experience, it can also be an invigorating and refreshing experience.

The recipient of the treatment will often report a 'balanced' feeling of peace and calm and will usually feel more alert and revitalised following a treatment.

Activity

Design a Marketing Plan for Indian Head Massage based on the following outline:

1 Description of the service to be offered (i.e. Indian Head Massage)

Include your unique selling points (USPs) and a full description of the service and how it can benefit others

2 Objectives of the marketing campaign

This could be to increase your client market, or to raise awareness of Indian Head Massage, etc

3 A profile of your intended client market

This is who you want to target and why you think they will pay for the service. Include as much information as possible based on what you have discovered about your potential clients (market questionnaires, interviews etc) Also include information on competitors, if applicable as this will help you to identify how much your potential clients are currently spending on a similar service.

4 Where you intend to offer the service (location)

Due to its portability, consider the different locations Indian Head Massage treatment may be offered in

5 Details of your SWOT analysis

(strengths, weaknesses, opportunities, threats)

6 Intended marketing strategies

Consider how you intend to advertise the service, what media you will use and often you will advertise.

Consider all the direct and indirect forms of marketing and promotions that will help your business succeed

Design a promotional leaflet for Indian Head Massage

Remember to allocate a budget for marketing activities and to plan the activities out over a period of time for maximum effect

BIBLIOGRAPHY AND FURTHER READING

Ashley, Martin
Massage – A career at your fingertips
Enterprise Publishing (1999)
ISBN 0-9644662-6-0

Bennett, Ruth
The Science of Beauty Therapy
Hodder & Stoughton (1995)
ISBN 0 340 63079 5

Burton, J.L.
Essentials of Dermatology
Churchill Livingstone (1985)
ISBN 0 443 03100 2

Caldwell, Diane
Marketing Campaigns
International Thomson Publishing (1998)
ISBN 1-86152-245-2

Cox, Gill and Dainow, Sheila
Making the Most of Yourself
Sheldon Press (1988)
ISBN 0-85969-478-X

Falloon, Val
How to Get More Clients
BPCC Wheatons Ltd, Exeter (1992)
ISBN 0 9513347 5 1

Fry, Lionel
Dermatology – An Illustrated Guide (Second Edition)
Update Publications Ltd
ISBN 0 906141 02 8

Gardner-Gordon, Joy
Pocket Guide to Chakras
Vibrational Healing Enterprises (1998)
ISBN 0-89594-949-0

Gaudin, Anthony J., Jones, Kenneth C.
Human Anatomy & Physiology
Harcourt Brace (1989)
ISBN 0-15-539705-2

Harland, Madeleine & Finn, Glen
Healthy Business – The Natural Practitioner's Guide to Success
Hyden House Ltd (1990)
ISBN 1 85623 000 7

Hole, J.W. Jr
Human Anatomy and Physiology
William C. Brown Publishers (1993)
ISBN 0-697-12271-9

Gill, Jit
Stress Survival Guide
HarperCollins Publishers (Collins Gem)
(1999)
ISBN 0 00 472321-X

Harish, Johari
Ancient Indian Massage – Traditional Massage Techniques Based on the Ayurveda
Munshiram Manoharlal Publishers Pvt. Ltd.
(1997 edition – originally published 1984)
ISBN 81-215-0008-7

MacKie, Rona M.
Clinical Dermatology
Oxford University Press (1991, reprinted 1993)
ISBN 0-19-261980-2

McGuinness, Helen
Anatomy & Physiology – Beauty Therapy Basics
Hodder & Stoughton Educational (1995)
ISBN 0 340 639436

Mernagh-Ward, Dawn and Cartwright, Jennifer
Good Practice in Salon Management
Stanley Thornes (1997)
ISBN 0-7487-2887-2

Mehta, Narendra
Indian Head Massage
Thorsons (1999)
ISBN 0 7225 3791 3

Oxford Concise Colour Medical Dictionary
Market House Books Ltd (1998)
Oxford University Press
ISBN 0-19-280085-X

Phillips, Carol
In the Bag – Selling in the Salon
Milady *Salon Ovations* (1995)
ISBN 1-56253-236-7

Premkumar, Kalyani
Pathology A to Z
VanPub Books (1996)
ISBN 0-9680730-0-X

Record, Matthew
Preparing a Business Plan
How to Books Ltd, Oxford (1998)
ISBN 1-85703-374-4

Sachs, Melanie
Ayurvedic Beauty Care
Lotus Press (1994)
ISBN 0914955-11X

Salvo, Susan G.
Massage Therapy – Principles & Practice
W.B. Saunders Company (1999)
ISBN 0-7216-7419-4

Sharamon, Shalila and Baginski, Bodo J.
The Chakra Handbook
Lotus Light Publications (1997)
ISBN 0-941524-85-X

Tortora and Grabowski
Principles of Anatomy and Physiology
Harper Collins (1992)
ISBN 0-06-046702-9

White, Dr Adrian
Stress and Anxiety (Help Yourself to Health)
Godsfield Press Ltd
ISBN 1-899434-38-0

Wilkinson, J.D. and Shaw, S.
Dermatology (A Colour Guide)
Churchill Livingstone
ISBN 0-443-05852-0

Williams, Sara
Lloyds Bank Small Business Guide
Penguin Books (1997)
ISBN 0-14-026836-7

INDEX